D1350868

Why Is it so Difficult to Die?

Second edition

Brian Nyatanga

Senior Lecturer, Institute of Health, Social Care and Psychology, University of Worcester

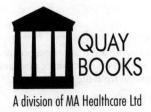

QUAY
BOOKS

A division of MA Healthcare Ltd

Quay Books Division, MA Healthcare Ltd, St Jude's Church, Dulwich Road, London
SE24 0PB

British Library Cataloguing-in-Publication Data
A catalogue record is available for this book

ISBN-10: 1 85642 370 0
ISBN-13: 978 1 85642 370 0

Printed by Ashford Colour Press Ltd, Gosport, Hants

Contents

Contents

To Priscilla, Pamela Lou, Neville and Lewin for their love and support always

To my parents who taught me so much about people

To my brother Lovemore for making me BELIEVE and realise what peace there may be in silence.

To colleagues and special partners who have unconditionally shared ideas, ideals and experiences, I am greatly indebted to you. Thank you all.

Contributors

Jean Bayliss
MA (Counselling), BA (Hons) PG Dip (Counselling in educational settings), ALAM Dip Life Coaching
After a background in education she was head of department in a further education college. At present she works as a counsellor and trainer, with a special interest in loss and grief. She is currently promoting clinical supervision to support practitioners in hospices, hospitals and trusts.

Simon Chippendale
MMedSc (Health Care Ethics), BSc (Hons), RGN, RNT, Cert Ed, Dip Pall Nursing
Simon Chippendale is a Senior Lecturer in Applied Health Sciences at the University of Gloucestershire where he is course leader for the Diploma in Palliative Care and Postgraduate Certificate in Advanced Practice (Health). As part of this role he works at Leckhampton Court Hospice, Cheltenham, for two days per week as Head of Education. He completed his Health Care Ethics Masters in Medical Science in 1996 at the University of Birmingham, and is currently a member of the National Council of Palliative Care Ethics Committee. Prior to his current post he has worked in palliative care education roles at a voluntary hospice, a national cancer charity and at the University of Birmingham.

Craig Gannon
MB, ChB, MSc, MRCGP, FRCP
Following his medical training in Birmingham Craig worked as a general practitioner before completing specialist training in palliative medicine. He now works as a consultant covering hospice, community and hospital settings. His interests include steroids and breakthrough pain, with a particular focus on clinical decision-making. As Specialty Training Committee chairman he had responsibilities for special registrar training across London (south) and Kent, Surrey and Sussex Deaneries since 2000.

Brian Nyatanga
MSc, PG Dip, Cert Ed, DIPSN, Dip Psychology, ENB 931, RGN
Brian Nyatanga is a Senior Lecturer at the University of Worcester. He has several years of clinical and educational experience in palliative care and has

written extensively on this area for the nursing press. His research interests are death anxiety and burnout and their impact on caring.

Hilde de Vocht
MSc Psychology

Hilde de Vocht is a Senior Lecturer at the Saxion Universities of Applied Sciences in the Netherlands. She is now working as a researcher in palliative care at the Expertise Centre Health & Social Care of Saxion Universities. Her research interests are problems and needs assessment and sexuality and intimacy in palliative care.

Acknowledgements

This second edition would not have been complete without new ideas and the support of a few people. You will see that there are new contributors and insights which I hope will enhance the book and make it more up to date for the reader. Firstly, in a more general way I would like to thank everyone involved for giving up their precious time to share their insights. However, a special mention and thanks must go to all the contributors of chapters in this book: Dr Craig Gannon, a dear friend and colleague of many years; Simon Chippendale, a colleague with a special passion for ethics of care; and Jean Bayliss, my previous Clinical Supervisor, mentor and professional guide. I owe a lot to Jean's belief in me and all her support and encouragement to take on the professional and educational challenges. A special thank you and warm welcome to a new contributor, Drs Hilde de Vocht for offering a Dutch perspective on euthanasia, and increasing the accuracy of our perception of the topic. I am truly grateful to you and your efforts in producing this work.

I would also like to thank Celia Robinson for her help with a new case study in Chapter 8, including the analysing using Kurt Lewin's theory. I wish to thank Dignity Funeral Services for help with up-to-date cost details of funerals in Chapter 10. These prices are specific to Dignity Funeral Services; therefore there may be slight discrepancies with other funeral services across the UK.

This second edition would not have been completed without the typing skills of my present secretary, Yulander Charles, and her calm influence. I am also grateful to my university for allowing me scholarly leave while writing this edition.

My penultimate appreciation is for my current professional mentor, Professor Joy Notter, for her support and encouragement particularly during difficult times. She has been instrumental in exposing me to useful networks and colleagues in the UK and abroad, and for that I thank her, and also for her inspiration and sound judgement.

Finally I would like to thank all the patients and their families and staff who shared their experiences and stories (often painful ones) with me during my clinical work, from which I gained a lot of knowledge and insight. I am even more grateful now that I am able to share it with others.

Brian Nyatanga
February 2008

Foreword I

Sir George Castledine

I am delighted to write the first foreword to Brian Nyatanga's second edition of his book, *Why is it so difficult to die?* with a focus in palliative care. There is no doubt that the first edition was a huge success and Brian and his colleagues are to be congratulated for achieving so much with such a concise piece of work.

The second edition has been fully revised and updated and there are now two parts and 12 chapters, with a final piece at the end of the book by Brian himself.

This is a book which will be very popular with those nurses who specialise in palliative care, but it is also essential reading for all nurses and health care professionals who want to know more about some of the key factors associated with death and dying. There is a genuine attempt by Brian and his colleagues to try to give some psychological explanations to the question 'Why is it so difficult to die?'. Brian leads the reader into the subjects within the book with a very easy and readable style which will appeal to a wide audience. The book is balanced in that it offers theoretical as well as practical aspects to death and dying

There are also some excellent contributions and a new chapter on dying by euthanasia by a new author from the Netherlands. This chapter offers clear insights into how the Netherlands manages euthanasia and assisted suicide requests.

I would strongly recommend this book to all those individuals who have an interest in this important subject and in doing so congratulate Brian and his team for not only maintaining the quality of their first edition but managing to improve and develop their work.

Sir George Castledine
Professor and Consultant of Nursing
Institute of Ageing and Health Birmingham and Sussex Healthcare UK

Foreword II

Dr Judy Dale FRCP

Be careful, then, and be gentle about death. For it is hard to die, it is difficult to go through the door, even when it opens
D. H. Lawrence, *All Soul's Day*

The six years since the publication of the first edition of Brian Nyatanga's book have seen great progress in developments towards better care for the dying.

The NHS Cancer Plan, National Service Frameworks and National Institute for Clinical Excellence (NICE) guidance all include strategies for improvement in palliative care services, including care of the dying. The Department of Health's 'Our Health, our Care, our Say' (February 2006) identified the need for investment and training to improve care at the end of life and the importance of choice for patients and carers.

The End of Life Care Programme 2007 aims to improve the quality of care at the end of life for all patients, and to enable more patients to live and die in the place of their choice. Best practice is encouraged in all settings through the use of the Gold Standards Framework and the Liverpool Care Pathway for the dying in the UK. Alongside these improvements in palliative and end of life care, there have been attempts through the House of Lords towards introducing assisted dying, leading potentially to the legalisation of euthanasia.

This book offers an excellent opportunity for professionals to develop their insight into issues around dying, particularly with the new chapter on the concept of death, dying and death anxiety, and the informative chapter by Hilde de Vocht about dying by euthanasia.

To be able to reach out to the dying, to communicate with them, and to understand their fears and anxieties, those caring for these patients must ask themselves the question 'Why is it so difficult to die?'.

Dr Judy Dale FRCP
Macmillan Consultant in Palliative Medicine
South Worcestershire, UK

Introduction

Palliative care is still relatively new to health, and is defined by the World Health Organization as:

> the total care of patients whose disease is no longer responsive to curative treatment and in which the control of pain, of other symptoms, and of the psychological, social and spiritual problems are paramount

The goal is to provide the best quality of life for patients and their families. Such care provision is most effective when carried out by a well-coordinated multi-professional team approach.

However, the World Health Organization has, in response to changing patient needs, and improved treatment options, revised the definition to:

> Palliative care is an approach that improves the quality of life of patients and their families facing the problems associated with life-threatening illness, through the prevention and relief of suffering by means of early identification and impeccable assessment and treatment of pain and other problems, physical, psychosocial and spiritual.

The different levels of palliative care provision (generalist, palliative care approach and specialist palliative care) are given and discussed briefly in Chapter 4.

The field of palliative care is charged with caring for all those affected by cancer. It is also now common practice to provide palliative care beyond cancer. It seems therefore that the challenge of providing palliative care is even greater now than it was a decade ago. It is no longer permissible, in palliative care terms, to focus only on the patient, excluding family and friends. The patient must be seen as part of the sum total of the family unit. This approach adds another dimension of challenge to providing palliative care, because of the diversity of family configurations in today's society. Finally, the biggest challenge is that most people continue to fear death, even though it is obvious that death is the only certainty in life. In a recent commentary (Nyatanga, 2005), I question the rationality of fearing death, since we are not consciously present when death occurs. Although most people agree with me that it is irrational to fear death, the truth remains that people still continue to fear death.

The question then is why this is still the case. A plausible explanation was offered by de Vocht in her response to the commentary, and this is worth reading, because it presents an interesting perspective. The different perceptions that people hold about death also reflect personal approaches, values and belief systems toward death itself. Since the first book was published, there does not seem to have been a real shift in attitudes towards death and dying, and therefore the question 'Why is it so difficult to die?' remains pertinent in this edition. It is my hope, and that of the contributors, that this second edition will provide additional information and thinking regarding death and dying. The new thinking might help readers to understand better the complex nature of the question we are posing. As more people understand why dying is difficult, they might begin to find ways of helping their patients negotiate their own death in their own preferred way.

Death is still viewed (particularly in the Western world) as a taboo topic, although there are now suggestions that this is no longer always the case. If this claim is accurate, and accepted, then the absence of this taboo should be more evident in palliative care setting, where death tends to occur more often than other settings. However, contrary to this, death is still not openly talked about by most dying people or their families. On the other hand, it is quite logical to suggest that the advent of palliative care itself has led to an increase in talking about death, but this is more so of health care professionals working within this setting.

A taboo, for purposes of clarification, and in the case of death, is something that is too 'horrible' to even talk or think about. In other words, it is something that is not mentioned openly in conversation. There is a simplistic view which suggests that not talking about death will somehow avert it, or make it go away. There is something about death that makes it so difficult to talk about and deal with the emotions it (death) provokes.

This second edition will attempt to offer a possible rationale for and discussion of why dying (as a process that leads to death) is difficult to negotiate. This book will, show using philosophical and psychological perspectives, why it is difficult for people to die, hence the title. More ground has already been covered in American literature on this topic, but we need to understand it from our own perspective; hence the focus of the book will be mainly British. This book takes a sensitive and honest approach to death and dying, as admittedly death can be a painful experience for most people. However, being sensitive should not be taken to mean weak, because this edition provides some challenging questions and arguments, some of which have not been discussed before. The book also aims to persuade readers to understand themselves first in the face of death and examine their own attitudes and beliefs, and perhaps begin to view death and its inevitability in a different way.

In the UK today, debates continue about whether to legalise euthanasia. While this move may be seen by proponents of euthanasia as affording dying people their final right and choice, it is not clear whether this alone will make dying an easier process. The new chapter in this book will give insights into dying in a country where euthanasia is already legalised. Such insights are useful and must be considered in relation to the British way of life, which is less liberal than in countries that practice euthanasia.

The book will explore the way a dying person may wish to negotiate his own passage from this life, therefore helping the health care professionals to understand this person more and hopefully provide better quality care. Chapter 8 offers practical information and suggestions about how to care for a dying person and the person's family. This part of the book is believed to be important in that it brings a balance between understanding the philosophical and psychological perspective of dying and what can be done in practice to help the dying person achieve a personally dignified death.

This book will be valuable reading for health care students and those undertaking continuing education programmes in palliative care.

The book is also aimed at those practitioners working in a variety of settings where death occurs. The Office of National Statistics has identified the different settings in which death occurs and published its figures in 1997. The places of death in England and Wales were identified thus: NHS hospitals had 53.3% of deaths, private nursing homes had 24.2% deaths, hospices accounted for 3.4% of deaths, and psychiatric hospitals had 0.8% of deaths. It was found that 10% of deaths occurred in non-NHS hospitals, with a further 8.4% dying in other establishments, including their own homes. These figures show that death tends to occur in almost every setting, and therefore this book will be useful reading for all the practitioners working in these areas.

However, a recent study by Davies *et al.* (2006) shows some changes in the numbers of deaths and places where the deaths occur. Table 1 shows the distribution of the deaths from three sources, and the point remains that hospitals still account for more deaths than any other setting. It is therefore more important that hospitals are well equipped (both in knowledge/skills and human resources) to afford every patient a unique death that reflects his individuality and humanhood. This book therefore remains relevant and applicable to these areas of care.

Table 1 Place and percentage of deaths. (Source: http://www.statistics.gov. uk/statbase/product.asp?vlnk=620; last accessed 1 March 2007)

	Hospital	Hospice	Own home	Nursing home
Field and James (1993)	54%	4%	23%	13%
Office for National Statistics (1997)	53.3%	3.4%	8.4% (to include other establishments)	24.2%
Davies *et al.* (2006)	44%	20%	30%	8%

Finally, it is important for the reader to appreciate the theoretical conceptual underpinnings of this book, without losing sight of the uniqueness of the individual who is dying, and who is central to our caring efforts.

Setting the scene

The first chapter is a brief overview of attitudes and their formation in general. This is followed by a close scrutiny on attitudes towards death between the 12th and 20th centuries. This will help to understand the transformation of attitudes to death that has taken place over time. This transformation is also arguably an indication of people's awareness of themselves and the degree of their individuality.

Chapter 2 is a philosophical exploration of death, dying and death anxiety. The philosophical dialogue is useful in our attempt to understand these concepts and how people may have different interpretations of them. The focus on death anxiety is an acknowledgement that the concept is elusive yet most troublesome among the dying, their relatives and the bereaved. This chapter will be of particular interest to academics, researchers and educators as it poses some challenging questions, arguments and explanations about the concept death. For example what part of the person actually dies, and is it the same person (identity-wise) who dies if they are constantly changing as they grow older or their condition deteriorates? Does identity affect our view of immortality?

Chapter 3 discusses the notion of a paradigm of death, and whether there is one. This will lead on to the exploration of a death system and the factors that shape it. This chapter provides an in-depth discussion of the philosophical and psycho-social and spiritual exposition of death. Examples are used to help explain complex philosophical arguments, and this is done to elucidate information and aid understanding while remaining reader-friendly. It will also be argued that death fear is common in our society and again a possible explanation as to its origin will ensue. A detailed discussion of the contexts of awareness based on the thinking of Glaser and Strauss is offered in order to explain this paradigm of death.

The following chapters, 4 and 5, focus on the perceived medicalisation of dying. Doctor Gannon, a consultant in palliative medicine, argues the ethical position taken by medicine in caring for all their patients. These chapters make some balanced arguments about the role of medicine in dying and death.

If we are not careful as professional carers, there is always a tendency to make patients dependent on us (for the wrong reasons) for all their needs. A pragmatic approach would be to enable patients to be self-reliant and to gain as much independence as their illness allows. It may be quite comforting to be needed by the patients we care for, as long as what we do does not stop patients regaining some of the lost control and independence caused by their illness.

Chapter 6 examines the ethical issues surrounding dying and death, offering a starting point of the principles of health ethics. Discussion centres on the issue of sanctity versus quality of life. This chapter also looks at dying ethically, thereby highlighting the dilemmas faced by dying patients, carers and professionals.

Chapter 7 is new and offers a different perspective on euthanasia. Although Dr de Vocht is based in The Netherlands (where euthanasia is legalised) the arguments offered are balanced and the reader should find this refreshing. The chapter offers detailed information on the notion of euthanasia and assisted suicide within The Netherlands. There are criteria for due care that each participating physician must adhere to if they are to avoid prosecution by the authorities. The ethical and moral positions for physicians and nurses participating in euthanasia are discussed.

Chapter 8 explores palliative care from a 'whole persons' perspective and offers practical ways of caring. A few examples are given to help reduce concepts, like the force-field analysis, to a useable level in practice. There is new material on spirituality and dying and how patients can be helped to express their needs at the different thresholds.

Chapter 9 offers an extra dimension in caring for the dying patient by exploring some cultural variations encountered by carers and professionals. This chapter utilises the factfiles already established for each cultural group. Use of such factfiles should not be taken as endorsement of the inherent stereotypical assumptions, but only as a way of offering a starting point for discussion on the topic. This chapter argues that there has been constant cultural modification (acculturation) and therefore it would be unfortunate to hold stereotypical views about the original culture, for example Muslim or Jewish. The argument centres on the pluralist society that we live in, and as a result cultures are bound to change, either through acculturation or enculturation. However, what is more important in this chapter is the consideration of what happens during dying and death, even for those cultures that have undergone acculturation. The chapter ends by offering suggestions on how to care for patients from different cultures.

Chapter 10 discusses the role of funerals and tries to answer the question: 'Are funerals and their rituals functional or dysfunctional for the bereaved?'. The idea of living with the dead is explored, showing how the dead may still keep a hold on the living through various ways. The role of obituaries is examined and so is that of funeral directors, again highlighting how death has become the business of others. This leads on to support the question posed by this book: 'Why is it so difficult to die in today's society?'. A brief section on children and funerals is included in this edition.

Chapter 11 discusses why it is now important to rethink about loss and grief and how to help the bereaved come to terms with their loss. Jean Bayliss looks at the staged theories and models of helping the bereaved cope with their grief. The shortcomings of these theories and models are highlighted, and then alternative ways of helping the bereaved are considered, moving away from focusing on grief as pathological, but as something that people can and should grow around. This chapter introduces new models and draws from research work carried out in New Zealand, The Netherlands and the United Kingdom on helping the bereaved come to terms with their loss at their own pace. The chapter offers a succinct summary of post-death activities. At the end of this chapter the reader will be left with new ideas, but for some inflexible practitioners this chapter may be a real challenge. There is a need to move away from working with order (staged theories and models), allowing chaos to prevail so that the bereaved can find their own order, without the time frames imposed by models.

The final word acts as a conclusion to the whole book, while highlighting some of the more poignant points that have emerged.

The contributors and I genuinely believe that this second edition is both informative and sensitive while discussing such a complex topic. The final goal for this book is to share ideas whilst developing a sense of proportion for the benefit of the dying patient and family. For professionals too, this book should help with their own perceptions of death and understanding some of the key challenges faced when patients are dying. It would be a great legacy to leave behind in palliative care if we can help to eradicate or minimise those aspects that make dying so difficult.

References

Davies, E., Linklater, K. M., Jack, R. H., Clark, L. and Moller, H. (2006) How is place of death changing and what affects it? *British Journal of Cancer*, **95**, 593–600.

Field, D. and James, N. (1993) Where and how people die. In: *The Future of Palliative Care* (ed. D. Clark). Open University Press, Buckingham.

Nyatanga, B. (2005) Is fear of death itself a rational preoccupation? *International Journal of Palliative Nursing*, **11**(12), 643–5.

de Vocht, H. (2006) Response Letter to Nyatanga's comment. *International Journal of Palliative Nursing*, **12**(4), 189.

WHO (1990) *Cancer Pain Relief and Palliative Care: Report of a WHO Expert Committee*. WHO, Geneva.

WHO (2002) http://www.who.int/cancer/palliative/definition/en/ (last accessed 10 March 2007)

Concepts in death and dying

CHAPTER I

Attitudes toward death

Brian Nyatanga

Introduction

The term *attitude* seems to be used loosely and in different settings so much that its meaning has become rather vague, as will be demonstrated in this chapter. It seems a logical starting point that, before exploring attitudes towards death, it may be worthwhile clarifying the term. You have probably heard people making comments such as: 'I don't like his attitude', 'He has got an attitude problem' or 'They will not tolerate that kind of attitude in this community'. We read about the attitude of Western countries towards certain issues, like abortion, human rights, corruption and suicide bombings, as inhumane or cowardly. We have also heard about some people in developing countries who, apparently, have no attitude at all towards AIDS or most of the above mentioned issues. When used in all these different ways the term *attitude* lacks a universal meaning. However, what seems to be universal in all the above examples is the reference made to viewpoints of either individuals or communities. Where a community is involved, this may refer to a collective viewpoint of that group of people. If we use the individual viewpoint, it can be seen that by not liking somebody else's attitude, this may suggest that he or she is not conforming to the expected norm. We must also consider that in such circumstances perhaps the problem lies with how a person interacts with another person's behaviour. For example it is possible that Pauline may find nose-picking in public disgusting, whereas Fiona may find nothing distasteful about that behaviour at all. It is obvious that Pauline's view (attitude) towards nose-picking is not favourable, but Fiona's attitude could be viewed as neutral, as she has not declared her support for the practice and neither does she find it disgusting.

Defining attitudes

The literature suggests that there is no single definition for 'attitude'. However, from all the definitions, including a sample given below, common elements emerge that would be useful to our understanding of attitudes. The first element is the way in which an individual believes and thinks about something, such as death or global warming. This mental or thought process is the **cognitive** dimension of an attitude. The second element is the **affective** dimension, which is how an individual feels about an issue or an object. In this case feelings are to do with how favourable or unfavourable someone or something is to the individual.

The final and common element is how the individual will respond or overtly react (the **behavioural** dimension) towards the situation or object. Secord and Backman (1964) claim that the behavioural component is based on both cognitive and affective elements. It is now generally accepted that attitudes help us to predict possible behaviour (Fishbein and Ajzen, 1980), albeit not that accurately.

Sample of definitions

An attitude is a mental and neural state of readiness, organised through experience, exerting a directive or dynamic influence upon the individual's responses to all objects and situations with which it is related. (Allport, 1935)

An attitude is a predisposition to act in a certain way towards some aspect of one's environment, including other people. (Mednick *et al.*, 1975)

Attitudes are likes and dislikes. (Bem, 1970)

Beliefs, values and attitude

Using the affective dimension of attitude, it can be seen that this is made up of values and beliefs held by an individual. In this blend, beliefs would represent the knowledge that a person has about a situation, in this case death, regardless of the actual accuracy or completeness of that knowledge. Such a belief may influence a person to link up the situation to some attribute. For example it is well known that Paris is linked with romance, hence Paris = romantic city, London = money, and death is often = suffering pain.

From a belief follows a value, which is what a person may view as desirable and worthwhile. Here there is an element of preference, which becomes a precursor to one's action. It follows therefore that values, unlike beliefs, which are non-evaluative and neutral, help a person to set standards to guide actions in order to achieve those values. According to Elms (1976), a combination of these two elements (beliefs and values) results in attitude. What must be clear at this point is that all these elements, including affective and cognitive aspects, are factually hypothetical constructs, as they cannot be observed or measured accurately, but must only be inferred from the observed behaviour or from listening to the other person's accounts/narratives. Behaviour itself is something that is learned through interacting with immediate family, peers, institutions and the social network. Morgan (1995) makes the point that people are socialised into an attitude by their culture. However, the attitude would remain intact and in its purest form provided that the original culture is not exposed to other cultures. Exposure would result in modification of the original culture, a process referred to by Devito (1992) as acculturation.

Development of attitudes

The understanding of attitudes is an important part of social psychology, perhaps because they (attitudes) are formed and influenced by families, social groups and institutions. This topic is vast and cannot be covered adequately here; therefore only a brief overview is intended. Attitudes develop from childhood experiences and through to adulthood and can affect a person's relationship with another. Children often have a naïve and simplistic approach to the unknown, such as death. In most cases children experience their first death through the 'loss' of an animal (family pet). The way in which such a death is handled depends mainly on parental influences, as parents tend to shape, primarily, children's attitudes. Most children tend to use their parents as points of references, and Morgan *et al.* (1979, p. 453) give an example of such reference: 'Mama tells me not to play with white boys' or 'Daddy says black people are lazy'. In this case, Morgan argues that there is a sizeable correlation between children and their parents' attitudes, albeit specific to religion and politics.

Although parental influence subsides as the children grow older, social influences become more evident in adolescence. Between the ages of 12 and 30 most attitudes stabilise (in other words they are formed) and Sears (1969) called this the **critical period**. This is also referred to as *crystallisation*, which commonly applies closely to adults, while the shaping of attitudes specifically affects the adolescence stage. An adolescent's attitude may vary, as it is not strongly held yet. As young adulthood approaches (i.e. moving into their twenties) most young people begin to make commitments. They may decide to vote in general elections, finish their education and start specialising in a particular career, or choose to get married. These commitments are made on the basis of the attitudes they hold, which tend to be crystallised, and may not change much afterwards.

Crystallisation of attitudes tends to create a need for consistency between attitudes and other information received. It is common to find people changing their attitudes in order to reduce any apparent discrepancy or disharmony. For example, any information that is not consistent within attitudes may demand two possible reactions so as to reduce the disharmony created:

- Explaining away (rationalising) that information and demonstrating intrinsically that it is not creating any dissonance
- Modifying or changing original attitudes to make them more favourable to the new information, thus reducing such dissonance.

Attitudes are also affected by peers, who are people of the same ilk, that is, age range and educational level, as those with whom we associate. Peers strongly influence the development of attitudes during adolescence. This is also a time when adolescents spent less time with parents, hence this 'see-saw effect'. Peers are powerful influences and adolescents see them as authorities and people they like to be around. They do things that are 'fun' and different from parental teaching.

Education, information and attitude development

Education tends to play a major part in attitude formation. However, it is worth noting that this also depends on how far one is educated. There is evidence to suggest that, in the main, people with more education hold liberal views (Sears 1969) and very often are of a high socio-economic status. The argument may be whether such liberal views make such people more accepting of their own death or not. They seem to be open minded with most things in life, but death poses a different challenge of immediate non-existence, and at times even the educated cannot rationalise the indiscriminate nature that death presents.

Information through exposure to television also contributes to attitude formation. In modern societies, television is the main influential medium in two ways:

- It plays a big part in weakening parental influence
- It portrays images and events vividly and explicitly to adolescents. Today, young people are more aware of what is happening around the world than they were two decades ago.

Religion and death attitude

Religion is thought to play a big part in relieving the fear of impending death (Malinowski, 1965). Indeed the relief of such fear can be applied in any crisis situation or experience encountered by human beings in their daily lives. Malinowski claims that religion functions to bring about a restoration of normality to the person experiencing the crisis. The question is what happens to those who do not believe in any religion (e.g. agnostics, who differ from atheists in that they feel that the concept of a God existing is too abstract even to discuss, and therefore their stance on the subject is silence).

But first we need to explore how religion can provide individuals with a means of dealing with crisis situations or phenomena. It is arguably plausible to suggest that death itself is often the phenomenon that calls for a religious intervention. At the same time, death is seen and accepted as the punishment for the sin committed by Adam and Eve in the Garden of Eden. Following after Adam and Eve, the individual is now born into sin and arguably is spiritually flawed. Religious individuals may find that religion provides them with more meaning and purpose in life, particularly in the last days of his life. For the religious, death may be seen as providing the passage (predetermined by a higher power) to eternity. The belief in a God or higher power becomes the influencing factor in providing equanimity for the dying person and his family.

There are other contrary views to this sacerdotal perspective. For example, Radcliffe-Brown (1965) claims that religion actually causes more anxiety in the dying person because of worrying about God's judgement, the possibility of going to hell and whether his life was lived according to the expectations of the religion or ritual. There are two points to make from Radcliffe-Brown's perspective. Firstly, it can be concluded that being religious could lead to dysfunctional consequences when faced with death, and secondly that non-religious or less religious individuals would experience less fear or anxiety about their own death. Both Malinowski and Radcliffe-Brown make valid points, but these should not be taken simplistically. Malinowski's theory focuses on the individual's perception of how religion functions for him, whereas Radcliffe-Brown bases his on society, in that society itself expects the dying to be anxious and fearful of their own death. When viewed like this, it can be seen that religion has an influence on ways of social integration. If it (religion) works for the individual, then it is also working for society.

On the other hand and if you subscribe to Radcliffe-Brown's perspective, the claim is that religion is in fact a catalyst that creates a sense of anxiety or fear, but this is positive because it helps to maintain the social structure of society.

Let us turn briefly to those who do not believe in God or a higher power, because they too negotiate their own dying. Arguably, agnostics have a belief that we probably do not fully understand and they utilise this in the face of death. Their meanings of death together with those of the religious tend to be socially ascribed. Death in itself is neither fearful nor non-fearful.

It is also true to suggest that in some cases religious people may find the threat of death so immense that they may be 'forced' to forsake their beliefs for something that may be the very opposite of their original beliefs. It is also plausible to suggest that the meanings ascribed to death in any given religion or culture are transmitted to individuals in the society through socialisation.

Death attitude

Having discussed general attitude, we should now focus the discussion on death attitude. The way one lives with dying and grieving forms one's attitude towards death. This attitude is three-dimensional, that is, cognitive, affective and behavioural, and therefore helps to present a complete picture of how the individual would deal with aspects and questions relating to death, dying and bereavement, and notions such as euthanasia.

Attitudes may involve feelings about dependency, pain, dignity, isolation, rejection, parting from loved ones, the afterlife and facing the unknown (Morgan, 1995). These feelings and reactions tend to be expressed in different ways by different people and at different times. Some people may talk very openly about their own death to the extent of making post-death arrangements, whilst others may avoid talking about it as if silence will make it not happen. Another way of explaining this death avoidance is to look at the different attitudes as a reflection of the different conceptions of what it is to be a person. This notion of existentialism also forms the basis of spirituality and the relationship of the person to his or her community, the world, God or a higher power. This concept of being a person will be discussed in detail in the following chapter. However, Morgan argues that even those who may appear to be open about death on a verbal level may be quite anxious subconsciously or at the fantasy level. As can be seen from different, and contemporary attitudes towards death, there are other ways of looking at death, dying and bereavement. However, Western society's attitude needs further exploration, not because it is dominant, but because it has been dominant in other areas of life (industrialisation, health and technology).

Aries (1974) postulated that attitudes to death over the centuries are indications of a person's awareness of himself or herself, and also of a degree of individuality. In his classification, Aries (1981) talks of four basic attitude orientations, which he calls 'Tamed death', 'Death of the self', 'Death of the other' and 'Death denied', which form the death system. A brief overview will be given here, but for the detailed account the reader is referred to Philippe Aries's books (Aries, 1974, 1981). The orientation of tamed death was dominant until the Middle Ages, when life was poor, nasty and short. It followed that one was constantly exposed to death and arguably became familiar with its presence. With such an abbreviated life, it was not common for young people to spend time, if any, preparing for adulthood. According to Morgan (1995) their courtships were short, relationships were limited and education was minimal.

According to Aries (1981) there was a shift of emphasis between 12th and 15th centuries, when the individual became aware of himself as distinct from the community. By making this distinction, it also meant that the individual fully ascribed to the death orientation of 'death of the self'. This was the realisation of the termination of one's life, one's personal death. Death became the last act of a personal drama, and at this point it was common to find tombs memorialising that life. Some tombs were placed in churches, and the different sizes probably symbolised the greatness of the person's life or memories being left behind.

In the 19th century, the above two orientations declined in favour of 'death of the other'. In this century life was viewed as having a meaning through relationships, (personal and intimate), and consequently death was viewed as a loss of that relationship. It can be argued that for close relationships to develop fully, privacy is a prerequisite, and if death then occurred in such relationships, it followed that it would no longer be a public event. In this context, death was no longer mourned as the loss to the community or as the end of life, but as the physical separation from a beloved one. The 20th century was seen as the period of death denied (Aries, 1981), where the death culture differed significantly from the preceding centuries. Here an understanding of the parameters of contemporary death attitudes becomes necessary, as they differ among cultures. The four major parameters to understand are: exposure to death, life expectancy, perceived control over forces of nature, and what it is to be a human being. These will be discussed in depth in the next chapter when the paradigm of death is discussed.

Concluding thoughts

[handwritten annotations: not happening all the time now, ppl living longer. Less contact with death → uncertainty, fear.]

It is now being argued that perhaps death is not so much denied, as claimed by Aries, but is simply unfamiliar to most people. With the advent of institutions such as hospices, hospitals and nursing homes where people die, it means that the family members may not always be exposed to death within that family. When death is viewed in this way it is being removed from the immediate family and witnessed by strangers who happen to be nursing and medical professionals. The argument that death has become unfamiliar would also suggest that people may not be comfortable with death, or simply may not know how to deal with its presence. If this is acceptable then it may also follow that people are fearful of death to the extent of not talking about it, because they lack familiarity with death. The other factor to consider in terms of death being unfamiliar is that people are now generally living longer than before. This lengthier/longer life expectancy is due to a variety of factors, including medical advances and technology, which have eradicated most deadly diseases, and a better informed public with a healthier lifestyle and improved diet choices. What this means is that most children growing up in families may not encounter death themselves until they are in their fifties, which means that they have to deal with death for the first time and also explain it to their own children. This is probably one of the reasons that make death so difficult to come to terms with.

On the other hand, recent discussions about end-of-life issues, with particular focus on priorities of care and place of death, may mean that more deaths will take place in patients' homes. End of life care requires an active and compassionate approach geared not only at supporting dying patients, but also comforting them as they live with their progressive life limiting conditions (Henry and Penner, 2007). If successful, this will reverse the picture painted above and help bring death back to the family home. The argument that remains is that such a move may be helpful in familiarising the whole family with death, but it might not make it any easier to talk about it than it is now. However, the fact that end-of-life discussions will place the patient at the centre and family members nearby may be one way of acknowledging the presence and inevitability of death.

This chapter has discussed the development of attitudes, and suggested that there is a sizeable correlation between the attitudes of children and their parents. If the parents have not formed an attitude towards death it may be even more difficult for the children to have theirs crystallised. There is, however, an avenue that could help with this apparent difficulty, when the influence of education to the development and formation of attitudes. Education should teach and discuss sensitively the concept of death, and this means that the teachers must feel comfortable and confident talking about death themselves. This kind of approach may not be a panacea, but is a step in the right direction, in that it allows discussion of a difficult topic to ensue in a controlled environment. Such an environment should also ensure that support (counselling) is available for those pupils who may find themselves perturbed by talking about death. It may also prompt pupils to ask their parents about death and dying, and this may be a welcome 'opening' for some parents, although others may not be comfortable answering such questions. I believe this is already happening with some families, but it needs to occur at a wider scale. This may even be beneficial to the dying if they can discuss openly their dying with the immediate family. The opportunity to bid farewell or apologise becomes a reality. One final word of caution is that attitude formation takes a long time to happen, and it takes equally long for attitude change to happen. What can be hoped for is to *affect* attitudes and leave it for the individual to respond.

References

Allport, G. W. (1935) Attitudes. In: *Handbook of Social Psychology* (ed. C. Murchison). Clark University Press, Boston.

Aries, P. (1974) *Western Attitudes toward Death. From the Middle Ages to the Present.* Marion Boyars, New York.

Aries, P. (1981) *The Hour of Our Death.* Knopf, New York.

Bem, D. J. (1970) *Beliefs, Attitudes and Human Affairs.* Brooks/Cole, Belmont, CA.

Devito, J. (1992) *The International Communication Handbook*, 6th edn. HarperCollins, New York.

Elms, A. C. (1976) *Attitudes.* Open University Press, Milton Keynes.

Fishbein, M. and Ajzen, I. (1980) *Understanding Attitudes and Predicting Social Behaviour.* Prentice-Hall, New Jersey.

Henry, C. and Penner , P. (2007) An Introduction to the NHS End-of-Life Care programme. *End of Life Care Journal*, **1**(1), 56–60.

Kastenbaum, R. (1992) *The Psychology of Death.* Springer, New York.

Malinowski, B. (1965) The role of magic and religion. In: *Reader in Comparative Religion: an Anthropological Approach* (eds. W. A. Lessa and E. Z. Vigt). Harper & Row, New York.

Mednick, M. T. S., Tangri, S. S. and Hoffman, L. W. (eds.) (1975) *Women and Achievement.* Hemisphere Publishing Corporation, New York.

Morgan, J. D. (1995) Living our dying and grieving: historical and cultural attitudes. In: *Dying. Facing the Facts*, 3rd edn (eds. H. Wass and R. A. Neimeyer). Taylor & Francis, Washington.

Morgan, C. T., King, R. A. and Robinson, N. M. (1979) *Introduction to Psychology*, 6th edn. McGraw-Hill, New York.

Nyatanga, B. (1997) Cultural issues in palliative care. *International Journal of Palliative Nursing*, **3**(4), 203–8.

Radcliffe-Brown, A. R. (1965) Taboo. In: *Reader in Comparative Religion: an Anthropological Approach* (eds. W. A. Lessa and E. Z. Vigt). Harper & Row, New York.

Sears, D. O. (1969) Political behaviour. In: *The Handbook of Social Psychology*, Vol. II (eds. G. Lindzey and E. Aronson). Addison-Wesley, Massachusetts.

Secord, P. F. And Backman, C. W. (1964) *Social Psychology*. McGraw-Hill, New York.

CHAPTER 2

The concepts of death, dying and death anxiety

Brian Nyatanga

This chapter starts with a brief discussion of death anxiety, highlighting its elusive nature in terms of a definition and triggers. A brief philosophical discussion of the concept of death is attempted. Such an attempt to explore the concept of death helps to establish a meaning of death. This exploration will show the significance of death and why its imminence provokes death anxiety in most human beings. Different types and theories of death anxiety are discussed, followed by an exploration of possible reasons why people are anxious about death. Factors capable of moderating how death anxiety is felt and experienced are also discussed. At the end of the chapter, a brief discussion is offered on how witnessing a patient's death experiences might impact on levels of death anxiety of health care professionals caring for dying patients.

Introduction

Most educators, researchers and practitioners alike teach about death anxiety. They teach how to ameliorate it and in some cases conduct research on it, and yet there is no consensus on what this notion is and what it means. Death anxiety is complex, as it has its base in both life and death. Without life, there would be no need to discuss death anxiety. In that case, in order to fully appreciate death anxiety, a brief understanding of life and death is crucial.

The complexity of death anxiety is further compounded by the interchangeable use of *anxiety* and *fear* as if these two terms were the same experiences. With this in mind, a distinction of the two terms will be attempted. More importantly, a definition of death anxiety will be offered which captures all the facets related to this notion. To do so a scrutiny of existing definitions will be conducted and the limitations of each highlighted before offering a most comprehensive definition of death anxiety.

The main point to consider here is whether caring for dying patients could provoke nurses to think about their own death and lead them to experience death anxiety. More important is the question of how experiencing high or low levels of death anxiety by palliative care nurses might affect the quality of care they deliver to dying patients. A review of the literature on death anxiety and nurses in palliative care settings will demonstrate how practitioners may be affected by increased death anxiety and fear and how this in turn may affect the care they give.

It is therefore important for palliative care nurses, educators and managers to develop policies that reflect how staff and patients may experience death anxiety, and what support is needed or appropriate for these professionals while they continue to provide this vital part of care. However, of paramount importance is an understanding of what death anxiety is, including how it may be triggered.

The elusive notion of death anxiety

The sensation of death anxiety is elusive, and how it affects the core of human existence is difficult to comprehend. The notion of death anxiety is arguably based on two main existential assumptions:

- life and death are interdependent, and
- death is a primordial source of anxiety (Langford, 2002)

Death is within us and although its physicality destroys. Heidegger (1962) claims that the idea of death saves us and somehow prompts us to 'shift' into a higher mode of existence. At this higher level, Heidegger argues that we move from forgetfulness of our being to a state of mindfulness. Although the shift in mental states can be useful, it also suggests that death is inevitably brought to the forefront of our thought processes, which in itself may result in increased levels of death anxiety.

On the other hand, despite the increased literature and discussion about death and dying (by, for example, Soren Kierkegaard, Martin Heidegger, Jean Paul Sartre, Simone de Beauvoir, Friedrich Nietzsche, Gabriel Marcel, Albert Camus and Edmund Husserl), death itself remains taboo in most Western countries (Kastenbaum, 1986; Neimeyer and Brunt, 1995; Nyatanga and de Vocht, 2006). A taboo would be regarded as something not openly talked about, therefore suggestive of a deep-seated anxiety about that phenomenon or object itself. The fact that death itself is the only certainty in life and yet it remains the greatest cause of anxiety. Somehow, some people still find it difficult to talk openly about death in general, let alone their own death. Even philosophers have not had consensus on why this happens or what makes death provoke so much anxiety in most people who have a concept of life. One of the causes of death anxiety was identified as the *unknown* nature of what lies beyond death (Parkes, 1978). The fact that death is guaranteed and yet unpredictable in its timing, making it indiscriminate, may offer a possible explanation for the cause of death anxiety. The fact that human knowledge and science have, up to now, failed to control or stop death completely makes death remain ill understood. When we fail to understand a phenomenon like death, there is a propensity to construct our own image of it. In this case, the image constructed media and held by most people tends to be largely negative or destructive, therefore inducing anxiety at the thought of it or witnessing another person's experiences of death.

Death anxiety can be viewed from different philosophical perspectives, and it is therefore worthwhile exploring some of these here. Indulging in such a philosophical dialogue is intended first to highlight the elusive nature of this concept, and second to bring about possible understanding which may lead to how best to research it. For practitioners, the challenge is how to respond and prevent it from developing amongst themselves while ameliorating it among patients. So far the discussion strongly suggests that death anxiety is inextricably linked with death; therefore, a discussion of the concept of death is important in order to fully understand death anxiety. In addition, the philosophical exploration of death anxiety might offer its epistemological basis. This may in turn make it easier to 'see' the possible interaction between death anxiety and burnout

After this discussion, a brief exploration of the distinction between 'anxiety' and 'fear' is offered, since these two entities are often used interchangeably, as if they are the same thing.

The concept of death

The possibility of death sub-consciously conjures up the greatest anxiety in human beings (Kierkegaard, 1844, 1849; Heidegger, 1962; Sartre, 1966). The anxiety is anchored upon the realisation of the possibility of not being (non-existence) in the world. The anxiety is worsened by the possibility of our nothingness, as well as the possibility of total disintegration of the self. This picture is further compounded by the possibility of grave uncertainties regarding events that may or may not occur beyond death.

What is death?

The term 'death' is ambiguous, as it has life as its precursor. For death to be possible, there has to be a life before it. However, the concept of life itself is not entirely clear. Additionally, 'the ending of life' is itself potentially ambiguous, as it is not clear when (at what precise moment) death actually occurs (Honderich, 2005; Kastenbaum, 2000). In dying, life is progressively extinguished, until finally it is gone (dead), in a process that stretches out over a period of time. This is true even if death is a threshold concept, that is, a sufficiently substantial extinction of life must occur before death takes place. This threshold concept applies to both chronic and sudden death. The only difference is the rate of extinction, which is quicker in sudden death. 'The ending of life' – hence 'death' – can refer either to this entire process, or solely to its very last part – the loss of the very last trace of life. Thus death can be a state, the process of extinction, or the denouement (final completion) of that process. Historical attempts to define death and the exact moment of death have been problematic, although physicians continue to certify death to a specific time. Table 2.1 shows some of the different types of definition of death. However, it could be emphasised (and is argued here) that, regardless of the definition and type of death it is, the advent of any death occurring is likely to provoke death anxiety. Here death is used to describe either a part or the whole of an organism ceasing to exist. The diversity here suggests various perceptions and understandings of the same thing – death.

If we were to reduce the ambiguity surrounding death, then death would be best viewed as the end of life in a biological (physiological) sense. This is marked by full cessation of the body's vital functions. This way of thinking led to death being defined as cessation of heartbeat and of breathing (Hinohara, 1948; Honderich, 2005). However, the advent of cardio-pulmonary resuscitation (CPR) and defibrillation techniques renders this definition inadequate. Successful resuscitation suggests that there may have been a 'temporary' death which is now reversed. If this was the case then it is impossible to say that death actually occurred, because once death has occurred it can not be reversed. Instead, something happened to cause temporary non-functioning of the bodily system, for example temporary cessation of cardiac or respiratory function. It seems somewhat indeterminate whether a temporary absence of life suffices for a death, or whether death entails a permanent loss of life. It may be useful, as a way of explaining this, to explore further Pallis and Harley's (1996) definition of brain stem cell death.

Pallis and Harley (1996) focus on two main capacities – the capacity for consciousness and the capacity to breathe spontaneously – both of which reside within the brainstem. The defence for the focus on the brainstem in defining human death is stated rather briefly. Consciousness is plainly central, since if

Table 2.1 Different definitions of death.

Type of death	Definition
Necrobiosis	Death of individual cells (except nerve cells) of an organism over a lifespan. New cells replace the dead cells in a continual process through a life span.
Necrosis	The death of many cells at once, which can result in the death of an organ or part of it. In medicine this is referred to as an 'infarction'.
Clinical death	Characterised by no breathing, no blood circulation and no brain activity. Clinical death begins with the onset of symptoms of death or cardiac arrest.
Brain death	Death caused by depriving the brain of oxygen continuously for 3 to 7 minutes. After that the brain can not be brought back to life again
Somatic death	A complete seizure: permanent and irreversible death of an organism. Such death in humans usually follows brain death as other organs rely on the brain to function, with the exception of artificial support.
Brain stem death	'A state in which there is irreversible loss of the capacity for consciousness combined with irreversible loss of the capacity to breathe spontaneously (and hence maintain a spontaneous heartbeat)' (Pallis and Harley, 1996, p. 3).
Cassell's Dictionary definition	Extinction of life, the act of dying. The state of being dead.

a human being is conscious then this is sufficient for their being alive. So too, as the definition indicates, is the *capacity* for consciousness. If a patient retains the capacity for conscious cognitive activity then they cannot be dead on Pallis and Harley's definition. The focus on the capacity to breathe spontaneously supposedly stems from the implied necessary relationship between breathing and life: if one has irreversibly lost the capacity to breathe, the definition claims, one is dead.

Pallis and Harley (1996, p. 3) suggest that the brain stem definition expresses 'philosophical, cultural and physiological concerns'. The significance of loss of the capacity for conscious thought is aligned with the departure of the 'conscious soul' . And the loss of the capacity to breathe signifies 'the permanent loss of "the breath of life"'. This understanding of death, it is suggested, 'is the implicit basis for British practice in diagnosing "brainstem death".

In summary, both the capacity for consciousness and the capacity to breathe are central components of the lay understanding of life. If one possesses either of these one is alive. When considering the question of when a person is dead, one is led to consideration of the presence or absence of these two key capacities. Pallis and Harley (1996) point out that both capacities lie within the brain stem. The capacity for consciousness lies in the ascending reticular activating system. And the capacity for breathing lies in the 'respiratory centre' within the brain system (Pallis and Harley, 1996, pp. 17–20). The presence or absence in a patient of the capacity for breathing can be determined by testing for this brain stem reflex activity, according to them. Out of all the definitions so far, this one seems more conclusive and convincing of what being dead entails, and is therefore persuasive for adoption in this thesis.

Religious perspective

According to some religious traditions, people's lives need not permanently end when their bodies break down. There are two main competing ideas about how life may continue. First, our physical demise could be temporary, since God might resurrect our bodies (restoring our mental life in so doing). Proponents of this idea of an afterlife sometimes apply 'death' to the breakdown of bodies.

Second, our lives may continue uninterrupted, assuming we are souls who survive the demise of the body. Proponents of this idea sometimes apply it to the soul's departure from the body, but both groups presumably acknowledge that 'death' would apply to the permanent ending of life. The suggestion that the soul departs the body concurs with the Cartesian dualism coined by the rationalist René Descartes (1596–1650) (Stokes, 2006). Although Descartes could not fully articulate the relationship of the two entities within the person, the question that follows from this is that of identity of the dead person or the other part (soul) that departs the body. However, this question is beyond the scope of this book. For now our attention turns to the distinction between anxiety and fear.

Anxiety and fear: the distinction

Most existentialists, following on from Kierkegaard's seminal writings, have attempted to address the notion of death anxiety. They have made enormous contribution toward its understanding, but without a general consensus on the meaning and epistemology of death anxiety. Up to now there remains a degree of ambiguity over the term *anxiety*. This ambiguity is further compounded by the interchangeable use of *anxiety* and *fear*, as if these two experiences were the same. As a starting point, it is worth clarifying (briefly) the distinction between these two terms.

The distinction between anxiety and fear, was best captured by May (1977) when he proposed a link between a threat to our basic fundamental values and the emergence of anxiety. However, this link alone seems weak, as one can feel anxiety and fear in response to the same threat or phenomenon. What makes the distinction is not the values involved, but a perception of an element of uncertainty (in the case of anxiety) and an actual danger (in the case of fear) (May, 1977). While fear has a clear object, that is, an imminent threat, anxiety does not; it is linked to uncertainty, which often leads to insecurity. In other words, what May is postulating is that, for anxiety to arise, our inner state feels insecure, which becomes more important than an external object threatening us. May (1977, p. 181) further elaborates that, in anxiety, it is the security pattern itself which is threatened, which then leads to feelings of anxiety.

Ontological anxiety

Ontology may be defined as the 'science of being' (Wyschogrod, 1954; cited in Honderich, 1995). The study of the form of things and their associations. Heidegger (Weston, 1994; Appignanesi, 2006) uses the concept of *dasein* (literally meaning 'to be there' in the world) to explore the ontology of human existence.

There are numerous commentators on the philosophy of death anxiety, for example, Heidegger (1962) 'the impossibility of further possibility', Kierkegaard (1947) 'the dread of non-being', Jaspers (1951) 'the fragility of being' and Tillich (1952) 'ontological anxiety'.

The fact that we live (being) is sufficient to create anxiety about how we preserve this state of our dynamic and creative self (Tillich, 1952; Heidegger, 1962). The tension is often between the state of our 'being', and the constant threat from the possibility of our non-being (Kierkegaard, 1947; Heidegger, 1962). This tension is what is being referred to as ontological anxiety (Kierkegaard, 1947; Tillich, 1952; Neimeyer, 1994). The threat of non-being is equated to or synonymous with fear of our own nothingness; therefore this can be seen as a cognitive (thought) process about what it is like to be nothing (Kierkegaard, 1947).

Ontological anxiety is provoked when there is threat on our being which is capable of turning us into non-being or extinction. According to Park (2001), there are some defining features of ontological anxiety:

- Generalised feeling of total threat to 'being', and this is viewed as free-floating anxiety;
- Anxiety which arises from within ourselves, with no identifiable cause;
- Permanent inner state of 'being'; that is utterly and constantly threatened; which often leads to insecurity
- Anxiety caused by threat to our collective values through our organs or system. If the organ is saved then death is postponed, and this prolongs our existence and reduces or prevents feelings of anxiety.

Defining death anxiety

It is well documented that there are definitional problems regarding death anxiety (Neimeyer and Brunt, 1995), but research studies on this notion continue to be undertaken. As already highlighted above, the interchangeable and sometimes careless use of the terms *anxiety* and *fear* has contributed to the current confusion and definitional difficulties of death anxiety. It seems the distinction between these two terms is not compellingly persuasive on conceptual or practical grounds. However, Neimeyer and Brunt (1995) claim that a distinction between fear and anxiety has often been made through the construction of instruments that assess them. For example, a questionnaire measuring death anxiety might ask about reactions to more abstract factors like apprehension about the state of non-being that death might represent (Neimeyer and Brunt, 1995). On the other hand, questionnaires measuring fear of death tend to focus on pain of dying (both physical and existential), and on individual reactions to death.

Other writers have tried to offer definitional clarity on death anxiety; for example, Thorson and Powell (1988) argue that death anxiety is best understood through its characteristics, which are multidimensional concerns such as denial of death, fear of death of self and others, avoidance of death, and a reluctance to interact with dying persons. Whilst this is useful in offering characteristics of death anxiety, it still fails to state what death anxiety itself is. It fails to discuss whether death anxiety is best defined as an emotion or a mood.

Lonetto and Templer (1986) have defined death anxiety as an 'unpleasant' emotional feeling upon the contemplation of one's own death. This definition, although useful, is restrictive, as death anxiety can also be provoked by witnessing or thinking of other people's death. However, one important distinction which can be inferred from this definition is that death anxiety is viewed as an emotion as opposed to a mood.

Tomer (1994) views death anxiety as the anxiety caused by the anticipation of the state in which one is dead. This definition, Tomer stresses, excludes related aspects, such as fear of dying or death of significant others. The exclusion of the death of significant others as provoking death anxiety makes this definition, like that of Lonetto and Templer, limited in that witnessing or contemplating of other people's deaths can provoke death anxiety.

Death anxiety from other perspectives

From a psychoanalytical perspective, Freud described death anxiety as a response to internal processes or external forces, having its roots in castration and separation anxiety (Freud, 1961). This view, however, is countered by a more behaviourist perspective that death anxiety is in fact a learned response of experiential origin; for example, Frankl (1963) describes this in *Man's Search for Meaning*. In view of the existential view and discussion earlier, viewing death anxiety as a learned response creates tension with the notion that our mere existence is itself enough to provoke death anxiety. The tension is thought to arise from the state of our being and the constant threat from the possibility of our non-being (see Heidegger, 1962).

Using a reductionist view of the universe (Sherman, 1997), the conventional assumption is to view death anxiety as a direct response to anticipating a death that comes as a result of a degenerative physical and mental process. The other view suggests death anxiety as a result of contemplating death as a form of mutilation and annihilation. The strong view of death as a destructive phenomenon or force has arguably created a predominantly negative interpretation, and this is what seems to provoke most death anxiety (Sherman, 1997).

Using the socio-cultural view, death anxiety relates to deprivation in the mother–child relationship (McCarthy, 1980) and might also have links to the person's cultural and historical background. According to Feifel (1959) and Neimeyer and Brunt (1995), the dimensions of death anxiety are fear of pain, punishment, loneliness and loss of control. Death anxiety can be viewed as related to the anxiety induced by the prospect of our own death, what happens after death and the fear of ceasing to be. These characteristics seem to be true of many patients approaching the final phase of their life.

Lonetto and Templer (1986) believe that sources of death anxiety are concerned with both the cognitive and emotional impact of dying and death; the anticipation of physical alterations; and awareness of the finite time between birth and death.

The above discourse demonstrates the complexity of defining death anxiety with its different perspectives. It also highlights key facets that encapsulate the notion of death anxiety. For Kierkegaard and Heidegger (Weston, 1994), death anxiety might ultimately be the fear of the possibility of not having any further existential possibilities.

> For the purposes of this chapter, death anxiety will be taken to mean: a disturbing emotion triggered by multi-faceted concerns and centering on the contemplation of the death of self and the death of others.

This definition does not suggest that this centering is exclusively on contemplation of death, but that this is *one* of the triggers. It is argued that death anxiety can be felt while caring for or witnessing the death and dying experiences of terminally ill palliative patients and not only close relations.

Readers of my previous publications (see Nyatanga and de Vocht, 2006) will note a slight shift in the definition. The current definition captures more closely than previously the essence of death anxiety, and therefore supersedes the earlier version.

It is tempting to argue for different types of death anxiety by claiming that one type is caused by concerns about one's own death and that another type is caused by concerns stemming from the deaths of others. As tempting as it may be, it does not seem plausible enough to be conclusive. However, what may be the most plausible argument here is accepting that the sources or triggers of death anxiety are different, one being indirect (i.e. stems from the death of others), but that this provokes them to think of their own death. In other words, the individual contemplates the death of others and then translates this into contemplation of their own death, and therefore can only feel one type of death anxiety.

Rosenbaum (1989) claims that most philosophers think that death anxiety is a reasonable emotion to experience, particularly if one concurs with the Aristotelian view that death is the most terrible of all things, and that it is even right and noble to be anxious about it.

On the other hand Plato's view was the opposite to this, when he wrote (in *The Apology*):

> No one knows whether death may not be the greatest of all blessings for man, yet men fear it as if they knew that it is the greatest of evils. And surely it is the most blameworthy ignorance to believe that one knows what one does not know

Toscani *et al.* (1991) describe the breakthroughs in medicine and how they have contributed to the postponement of death by prolonging the period of dying. This view arguably suggests that death is not always welcome, and therefore different measures are taken to try to avoid or prolong its occurrence.

Toscani *et al.* claim that death, which was once viewed as a natural event, is now associated with a 'pathological' condition which must be faced aggressively using techniques which often interfere with and indefinitely delay the necessary biological process that lead to death.

Despite the differences in conceptualisations about death, Templer (1970), Thorson and Powell (1988), and recently Abdel-Khalek (2002) developed a death anxiety measurement scale which reflected on a wide range of life experiences covering the act of dying, the finality of death, corpses and burial. It is true that most things in life are capable of inducing an emotional reaction, but for the purposes of this discussion only death-related emotions lead to the experience of death anxiety. The death or dying processes that one is exposed to do not have to be of self, but can include close friends, family or others such as dying patients.

The point to consider here is whether caring for dying patients could provoke nurses to think about their own death and lead them to experience death anxiety. More important is the question of how experiencing high or low levels of death anxiety by palliative care nurses might affect the quality of care delivered to dying patients.

It is therefore important for palliative care nurses, educators and managers to teach and develop policies that reflect how staff and patients may experience death anxiety and what support is needed or appropriate for such professionals while they continue to provide this vital part of care.

Why people are anxious about death

Although the exploration so far in this chapter helps with the understanding of the concept of death anxiety, it does not tell us why death is not always welcome, to the extent of being feared. Two main questions arise as we attempt to answer why people continue to be anxious about death:

■ Is death bad for those who die?

and

■ Does death harm the dead?

(Both questions being subsumed in the sense of lack of specific knowledge)

In an attempt to answer these questions, we need to consider when death occurs (the moment of death) in relation to the dying person's consciousness, and how life is viewed before death occurs. The actual moment of death is not as clear cut as those certifying a death seem to make us believe. This question is beyond the scope of this chapter, but work on this is under way and will be published separately in due course.

The above questions need considering in relation to a palliative carer's consciousness and preview of dying and death.

First, is death bad for those who die? To consider something 'bad' suggests that there must be something 'good' with which to compare it. In this case the suggestion is that death brings an end to life, which has to be seen as a good thing. All things being equal, what ends good things is bad. However, the same conclusion would be limited if one felt that life was not good, instead death might be seen as a welcome end to a bad life.

The second question is 'Does death harm the dead?'. To answer this, we consider the symmetry argument by Lucretius (1951). Lucretius, an Epicurean poet, argued that no one fears the time before which one existed. In other words no one is afraid of prenatal existence, because one is not aware of it. In this context, the time before which one existed (pre-birth) is relatively similar to one's future non-existence (death). The central argument is that one cannot be affected negatively by the two non-existences, as one has no experience of either of them. Lucretius makes one further point by suggesting that nobody justifiably believes that one's future non-existence is relatively different from one's prenatal non-existence. Therefore, it is not reasonable now to fear one's future non-existence, one's being dead and one's death. From this analysis, it is therefore irrational for death to then harm the dead.

So death, the most frightening of all bad things, is nothing to be feared and the rationale is given simply as follows:

> When we exist, death is not yet present; and
> When death is present we do not exist.
> In this analogy, death is neither relevant to the living nor the dead.

To recap the point made earlier about being affected negatively by either prenatal or post-death existence: it becomes crucial, if one is to refute the assertion of the symmetry argument, that proof be established of the difference between the two extreme existences. This observation was made by Nagel (1970), who argued that there is a difference between prenatal and posthumous non-existence. His argument is simply that the time after a person's death is a time of which his death deprives him. It is a time in which, had he not died, he would be alive. Therefore any death entails the loss of some life that its victim (the dead) would have led had he not died. It can be concluded here that Nagel is implicitly suggesting that we cannot say something similar about pre-birth, hence he exposes the asymmetry between prenatal and posthumous non-existence. However, what he does not refute is that the dead person has no concrete conception of this time he has been deprived of once he is dead. In that case Lucretius's argument seems to be more persuasive, but only at a rational philosophical level, because in reality people still fear death (Nyatanga, 2005; Lester, 1994). The fact that rationality cannot help us explain why people continue to fear death does not mean that people should not fear death. Instead, other ways of explaining and understanding the basis and triggers of the fear should be sought.

Interesting and forceful though these arguments are, their relevance may be somewhat abstruse to palliative nurses, who are likely to be more concerned with the practical aspects of death and death anxiety.

What exactly do people fear when they fear death?

In order to answer this question, a further question needs to be asked: is death a certainty or an uncertainty in one's life? If death is perceived as an uncertainty, then it is justifiable for most people to fear it. There is also the element of 'the unknown' (Parkes, 1978) which lies beyond death and which troubles many people, particularly those who do not believe in life after death. On the other hand, if death was perceived as a certainty, it would not be justifiable and rational to fear it unless it was prematurely present, thereby disrupting one's future goals and aspirations. However, there is another argument which exonerates death from causing fear and places it on the process of dying itself as the real sources of the fear.

It is argued that it is not death itself that people fear, but what is associated with its arrival or presence. It is more the process of dying and the impact of death than death itself that people fear. The dying process can often be long-protracted and include pain, suffering, fear and loneliness. Death causes a multitude of losses and at different levels of human existence, e.g. social, psychological, emotional, physical and spiritual. Death indiscriminately robs dying people and the bereaved of control over their lives and aspirations. Some people believe in an afterlife and may fear death because it may not deliver the afterlife they were anticipating. The fear comes from not knowing what post-death outcomes will be. There are several reasons for this fear, one of which is premature death, and hence the dead person is not well prepared to enter (or be entered) into an afterlife. However, the problem of talking about a premature death suggests that there might be an acceptable point in life when death is welcome (mature death). It is true that even in the 'very old', death is not always accepted. It is difficult to reject the notion of an afterlife, since so many people report the experience (Williams, 2005). The question to ask here is: 'If there is an afterlife, what type is it going to be, heavenly or hellish?'. Williams (2005) believes in the principle that life is what you make it and he is convinced that the afterlife will be based on the same thinking. He gives an example: we can kill and end up in prison or we can do good things and live contentedly. Williams believes this principle belongs to hell and heaven, but for us what is even more important to consider is that if fear of death is justifiable, it would have to be the fear of going to hell.

The next section focuses on types of death anxiety followed by a discussion on the early theories of death anxiety and how they have shaped our understanding of this phenomenon.

Types of death anxiety

As already noted earlier, people are different and therefore their experiences of death anxiety are bound to differ. However, Langs (1997) claims that death anxiety is prompted by any traumatic event, and that it can register and operate entirely outside of awareness. Langs (2004, 1997) further concludes that there are three classifications of death anxiety: predatory, predation and existential anxiety.

Predatory death anxiety is evoked by dangerous situations (traumas) that put the individual at risk and are seen as threatening survival. These traumas can be physical, psychological or both in nature. The presence of this death anxiety mobilises the individual's defensive resources, leading to 'fight or flight' response to combat or escape the danger. The responses, Langs claims, can take physical or cognitive forms and include both conscious and unconscious processing and modes of adapting (Langs, 2004).

Predation death anxiety arises when an individual harms (either physically or mentally) other human beings. The advent of this anxiety often involves unconscious rather than conscious realisation and processing (Langs, 2004). However, the primary reaction to this anxiety is that of conscious and unconscious guilt. This feeling of guilt often leads to self-punitive decisions and actions by the perpetrator.

Existential death anxiety is probably the most powerful of anxieties and is well entrenched in our human existence. It is activated in humans with a definitive, conscious awareness and anticipation of the inevitability of the individual's demise (Langs, 2004). The individual's ability to anticipate the future and its possibilities is threatened by the possibility of non-existence. According to Langs, humans defend against this type of death anxiety through denial, often effected via a wide range of mental mechanisms and physical actions. While limited use of denial tends to be adaptive, its use is often excessive, which often proves emotionally costly in the long term (Langs, 2004; Langs, 1997).

Theories of death anxiety

Early thinking about death anxiety was influenced by two main theories, the first of which is due to Sigmund Freud (1856–1939); specifically his works published in 1953, well after his death, recognized that people sometimes expressed fears of death. These thanatophobic expressions (as Freud suggested) were a disguise of deeper sources of anxiety, and not death and qualified his reservations by writing (Freud, 1953):

> Our death is indeed unimaginable, and whenever we make the attempt to imagine it we only survive as spectators... at the bottom nobody believes in his own death, or to put the same thing in a different way, in the unconscious every one is convinced of his own immortality.

According to Freud, the unconscious mind does not deal with the passage of time, and does not register that this life will one day come to an end. He also argues, like many other writers, that one cannot fear death because one has never died. This assertion can only be true on a rational/logical basis, because the reality is that people continue to fear death. Freud's explanation of fear of death is that such fear is focused on unresolved childhood conflicts, which are too painful to acknowledge and discuss openly. It seems Freud was basically reducing fear of death to some neurotic underpinning, and this remained so until Becker's existential theory of 1973.

Becker (1973) postulated that not only is death anxiety real, it is most people's profound source of concern. Becker claimed that most people's daily behaviour consists of attempts to deny death and thereby keep death anxiety in check. However, it would be difficult to control one's anxiety if one were constantly exposed to reminders of their vulnerability. This example can be related to palliative nurses who are constantly being exposed (through caring) to other people's dying experiences. Becker argued that it was the function of society to put in place mechanisms that would strengthen the individual's defences against death anxiety.

Other approaches, like terror management theory (TMT), which suggest a way of managing death anxiety, were introduced in the late 20th century. Terror management theory (Greenberg *et al.*, 2004) supports the view that people who feel better about themselves also reported having less death-related anxiety. To feel better about themselves suggests strong high self-esteem, which, along with other constructs like personality hardiness, locus of control, self-efficacy and others, acts as a buffer against death anxiety. Enhanced self-esteem is thought to be one of two main mechanisms people use to cope with mortality threats (Smieja, 2006). The other mechanism is worldview confirmation, which is based on symbolic construction that gives order to and meaning of life (Smieja, 2006).

Another theory, regret theory, was proposed by Tomer and Eliason (1996). This theory is closely related to the ideas being discussed in this chapter, and therefore more discussion will be dedicated to it here. Regret theory puts emphasis on how people evaluate the quality or worth of their lives. The prospect of death is likely to make people more anxious if they feel that they have not and cannot accomplish something 'good' or positive in life. People might torment themselves with regrets over past failures, missed opportunities and future achievements that will now never be possible. Tomer and Eliason have proposed an integrative model of death anxiety to show how regret leads to anxiety. The model has three main antecedents of death anxiety, namely past-related regret, future-related regret and meaningfulness of death. The two regret-oriented determinants are induced by contemplation of one's death. Past-related regret is based on the perception of not having fulfilled basic aspirations in life. Future-related regret refers to the perceived inability to fulfil basic goals in the future. The third antecedent, meaningfulness of death, refers to the individual's perception of death as negative or positive, that is, making sense of it or not. From this model one will experience death anxiety if one has regrets and/or perceives death as meaningless. According to this model, the three determinants of death anxiety are related to the extent to which the individual contemplates his mortality, thereby making death salient. It can be argued that this model seems to closely reflect most people's perceptions of death and its impact on them; hence its choice here for elaboration. This model places the individual in the centre of a 'life journey' that most people travel, where they have a past with its joys and regrets/missed opportunities, the present with current activities and a future with aspirations and opportunities to be fulfilled. However, this also suggests that the model is not perfect, and this will be highlighted through the discussion below. Figure 2.1 is an illustration of this model as proposed by Tomer and Eliason. In addition to the three determinants, the coping process of the individual plays a part in the outcome of death anxiety. Although not clearly stated here, the coping process would logically refer to the dying process as opposed to death itself. The individual's beliefs about the self and the world are also key considerations, as they both feed into the meaningfulness of death, and therefore are antecedents.

From this model it is not clear what constitutes beliefs about self. It can be argued that these beliefs are based on positive self-esteem, self-efficacy and self-worth. The meaningfulness of death needs expanding on to make it clear that such a meaning can be both positive and negative. The type of meaning-

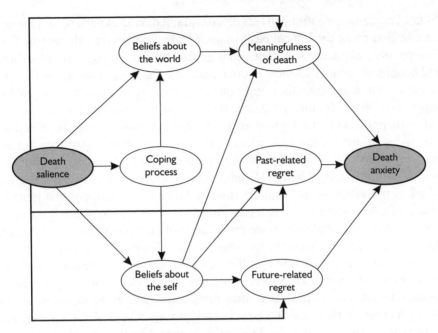

Figure 2.1 A model of death anxiety (Tomer and Eliason, 1996).

fulness and a sense of self will affect and impact the level of death anxiety experienced. Death anxiety need not always or exclusively be dependent upon regret. A direct link to a person's sense of self may be a more instructive area to explore. Instead of future-related regret, a threat to future aspirations may cause death anxiety. Past-related regret is better expressed as meaning of life at present and whether this is negative or positive.

There are other factors that can be seen as sources of death anxiety. For example, for some people, happiness is arguably the most sought-after possession in life, and therefore everything (work, relationships and business) is ultimately geared to achieving happiness. The future and meaningfulness of life will also be discussed to show how they too are sources of death anxiety.

Sources of death anxiety

Happiness as a source of death anxiety

The fact that death is probably the only certainty in life and yet most people continue to fear it seems to have no justifiable and logical basis (Williams,

2005). People who continue to fear death without having experienced it prompt the question about the logical basis of such fear, and what exactly they do fear. One possible explanation is that death as we know it deprives life of its joys and happiness, goals that most people aspire to. Death disrupts the possibility of further life and the realisation of one's aspirations and desires. The goal of happiness and its significance can be traced back to Aristotle, who maintained that it (happiness) is the highest good; the highest good is what is valued for our sake and not for the sake of anything else. However, using the doctrine from Epicurus (341–270 BC) and the Epicureans, happiness alone is not sufficient as a final state of being. Happiness is therefore associated with pleasure which is perceived as the ultimate state of exaltation. There are two types of pleasure, moving and static, and pleasure itself is also seen as satisfying one's desires. The moving pleasures are associated with the process of satisfying the desire, e.g. eating a cheeseburger when one is hungry. The actual process of eating would involve an active titillation of the senses of taste and associated physiology, which would in turn create the feeling that most people refer to as pleasure. It then follows that after the desires have been satisfied, maybe after a burger or two, and the person feels no need or desire for more, this state is itself pleasurable; the Epicureans referred to this as static pleasure, which also happens to be the best pleasure one can achieve. It is important to try to apply this idea of pleasure at different levels and not just the physical, as in the example. Psychological pleasures can encompass fond memories or regret over past mistakes or omissions, whilst fostering future confidence of pleasures to occur.

This is important to understand, because the Epicureans strongly believed that all the happiness and pleasures can be destroyed by anxiety about the future, especially that of death. If this destruction was to be avoided, it is therefore imperative to banish fear about the future and death. Their belief was to face the future with confidence that one's desires will be met, which will lead to a state of ataraxia (total tranquillity) of mind. Given the above position, and the advent of cancer and other life-limiting diseases, health care professionals are aware that death is a reality. They may therefore experience anxieties about their own mortality, no matter how irrational this may be. The point to recap here is that death makes life impossible; it brings a 'good' thing to a close. As Frances Kamm (1998) emphasised, we do not want our lives to be all over with.

The future as a source of death anxiety

The future and all its potential is based on our ability to exist. According to Parfit, we have a far-reaching bias extending to goods in general: we prefer that any good things, not just pleasures, be in our future, and that bad things, if they happen at all, be in our past (Parfit, 1984). Parfit argues that if we take this extensive bias for granted, we can explain why it is rational to deplore death more than we do our not having always existed: the former, not the latter, deprives us of good things in the future. Death or being dead is the only thing certain of denying us future desires. Having knowledge of this possibility is enough incentive or motivation to do everything possible to prevent death. The thought that death may not be prevented might reasonably be the source of anxiety, and in this death-related context it makes perfect sense for this type of anxiety to be termed death anxiety.

Whether or not we have the extensive bias described by Parfit, it is true that the accumulation of life and pleasure, and the passive contemplation thereof, are not our only interests. We also have active, forward-looking goals and concerns. Engaging in such pursuits has its own value; for many of us, these pursuits, and not passive interests, are central to our identities. However, we cannot make and pursue plans for our past. We must project our plans (our self-realisation) into the future, which explains our bias towards future desires. It is not irrational to prefer that our lives (existence) be extended into the future rather than the past, if for no other reason than this: only the former makes our existing forward-looking pursuits possible. It is not irrational to prefer not to be at the end of our lives, unable to shape them further, and limited to reminiscing about days gone by. It can be seen from this discussion that anything threatening our future pursuits can easily provoke anxiety specific to our future non-existence, hence death anxiety.

Anxiety related to meaninglessness (or absurdity)

This anxiety is well known from existentialist and postmodern language. It derives from the lack of (a) a feeling of mastery of one's existence; and (b) the experience of meaningfulness (dedication, vitality). Both sides are closely connected. This anxiety refers to what Kierkegaard called the possibility of being forgotten or lost in the universe (Kierkegaard, 1844).

The concept of death anxiety again does not primarily refer to the fact of one's (own) death or to the process of dying. On the contrary, it refers to anxiety as an expression of the openness toward one's finitude (finiteness) and mortality. It consists of honestly and authentically facing the possibility of one's own death. Anxiety, conceived in this way, is closely connected with life itself. Table 2.2 gives a breakdown of the different types of anxieties, themes and structures underlying their input in one's life. The last one in the list refers to death anxiety, with its theme in non-existence.

Table 2.2 Typology of basic anxieties, their themes and underlying structure.

Type	Theme	Structure
Anxiety related to loss of structure	Chaos	Identity–self relationship
Anxiety related to existence as such	Factual	Capacity to shape one's existence
Anxiety related to lack of safety	Vulnerability	Physical protection
Anxiety related to unconnectedness	Isolation	Affective connectedness
Anxiety related to doubt and incapacity to choose	Irrevocability or lack of control	Historical; capacity to believe and make choices
Anxiety related to meaninglessness	Absurdity	Mastery; capacity to entrust
Anxiety related to death	Non-existence	Openness; capacity to transcend

It is clear from this typology that anxiety related to death is duly identified as death anxiety. What is of importance is the theme from which it stems – that of non-existence – and which justifies the suitability of the definition of death anxiety proposed earlier in this chapter. In a sense death anxiety and its impact can be modified by other influences or variables. Death anxiety is seen as a dependent variable being affected by independent variables such as age and sex. Below a few variables that modify death anxiety are considered.

Variables affecting death anxiety

The experience of death anxiety can be modified, and in some cases prevented by various variables. These include age, sex, ego integrity, psychosocial maturity (Belsky, 1999; Erickson, 1982; Rasmussen and Brems, 1996), religiosity (Duff and Hong, 1995), locus of control (Hickson *et al.*, 1988), purpose in life and the environment (Goebel and Boeck, 1987). These are not exhaustive, but form the basis for the discussion below. The impact of these variables on death anxiety has been demonstrated in different research studies and will now be discussed.

Age and death anxiety

Age has been studied at length (Rasmussen and Brems, 1996; Erickson, 1982; Erickson, 1963; Belsky, 1999). Initial theories, not surprisingly, have hypothesised that as people grow older and closer to death, they would have more anxiety about death (Belsky, 1999). The assertion here is that with old age (that is, number of years), the possibility of death becomes closer and more realistic. It also suggests that life is viewed as a good thing, with more desires and aspirations to fulfil. Age was, and still is, a factor that can determine the levels of death anxiety in most individuals. However, age alone might not be a sufficient determinant of how one experiences or feels death anxiety. According to reports by Rasmussen and Brems (1996) and Erickson (1982, 1963), age should therefore be considered together with the maturity of the individual together with his ego integrity.

Ego integrity and death anxiety

Erickson's theory of Psychosocial Development suggests there are eight stages of human development. Each stage is perceived as an emerging task or challenge whose achievement or lack of it affects the next stage (Erickson, 1982). Erickson's theory has also been known as the Epigenetic Theory of human development. Epigenetic in this context means 'upon emergence'. Thus Erickson postulates that as people go through stages of life, they encounter developmental tasks or challenges. Of interest in the context of death anxiety is the last stage of the theory which focuses on integrity versus despair. From the age of 50 onwards, people reach this final (eighth) stage and may attain 'ego integrity'. Ego integrity denotes the ability to reflect on one's strengths and weaknesses in life with a sense of acceptance and dignity. Despair, on the other hand, denotes regrets and anxiety about aspects of one's existence. For example, if a person reviews his or her life and concludes that it has been a series of missed opportunities, this suggests that integrity has not been attained (Erickson, 1982; Belsky, 1999). Drawing from Erickson's theory, older adults who attain ego integrity should experience lower levels of death anxiety. It is also possible that such adults might not experience any anxiety at all given the degree of their ego integrity if it is characterised by fulfilment and contentedness, just to name a couple aspects. In summary, ego integrity can influence how one interacts and copes with life events such as stress. Stress often leads to burnout, and this notion is not being discussed here. However, it should be considered for future publication to show the link between anxiety and burnout among those who care for dying patients.

Psychosocial maturity and death anxiety

In another study examining the relationship between death anxiety and age, Rasmussen and Brems (1996) argued that the differences and discrepancies in death anxiety might be due to a third variable, that of psychosocial maturity. Psychosocial maturity suggests that individuals who are psychologically and socially contented and balanced can function effectively in the face of death. Rasmussen hypothesised that a person with high psychosocial maturity would have less death anxiety. She further made the assertion that psychosocial maturity was a better and stronger indicator of death anxiety than age alone. Rasmussen's findings suggest that both age and psychosocial maturity are inversely related to death anxiety.

Other studies have found no differences between age and death anxiety measurements. Goebel and Boeck (1987) found no relationship between death anxiety and age. However, considering that the participants used in this study were over 70 years of age, the chances of them having developed a high level of ego integrity are equally high. Higher levels of ego integrity would suggest that such individuals will experience less death anxiety. However, the only logical conclusion from Goebel and Boeck's study would be that, although older adults experience less death anxiety, age is not a significant factor in determining the degree of death anxiety felt in late adulthood.

A sense of purposefulness in life and death anxiety

A study by Quinn and Reznikoff (1985) explored the relationship between death anxiety and a sense of purposefulness in life and perceptions of time. According to Quinn and Reznikoff, people with high levels of death anxiety had a lowered sense of purposefulness to their lives. However, the same people had an increased sensitivity to time moving on. The point here might be that people who are less focussed on the future and their contribution to it would feel less death anxiety. Quinn and Reznikoff concluded that the older adult's decreased awareness of the future may, in fact, be a healthy way of responding to death and helping to lower death anxiety.

The above studies have focused on older adults and the relationship with death anxiety. There are no studies found that have been conducted to measure death anxiety among younger adults. It is worth pointing out here that, in general, people feel more emotive about a young person's death than that of an elderly person (Belsky, 1999). Therefore understanding the impact of a young death on health care professionals' levels of death anxiety would be important. One probable explanation of the impact of death on different age groups relates to the concept of an elderly person having had the opportunity to live a full and fulfilling life. It can be argued that for a young person, his dying would probably have denied him the opportunity of a complete fulfilment of life.

The environment and death anxiety

Some studies have tried to measure the impact of where people live and levels of death anxiety. One study by Goebel and Boeck (1987) examined the effects of different types of dwellings and death anxiety. They concluded that ego integrity was a significant factor affecting the impact of living environment on death anxiety. One specific finding was that people with low ego integrity living in nursing homes reported higher levels of death anxiety than those with low ego integrity but living in an apartment complex. In contrast, there was no difference in death anxiety in those with high ego integrity individuals living in either environment.

From this, there may be another factor to consider, that is, the level of control that people are able to exert on the environment. It can be argued that the higher the ego integrity individuals have, the greater their tendency to have a sense of control within themselves, so that they are better able to deal with external factors such as those found in most nursing homes. On the other hand, people with low ego integrity have a limited sense of control within themselves and on the environment. It can be concluded that such individuals may experience greater stress, leading to high levels of death anxiety.

Locus of control and death anxiety

Locus of control comprises two dimensions, internal and external. External locus of control attributes events and achievements to powerful outside forces and chance, which people have no control over. On the other hand internal locus of control attributes events and achievements to one's own ability, effort and determination (Rotter *et al.*, 1962). A study by Hickson *et al.* (1988) examined the relationship of locus of control to life satisfaction and death anxiety. Their findings concluded that an older adult's sense of control affects life satisfaction, which in turn affects death anxiety. In other words, they found an inverse relationship between life satisfaction and death anxiety. Berman and Hays (1973) report in their study with 300 college students that no relationship was found between external locus of control and death anxiety.

Religiosity and death anxiety

Religiosity has been of interest to researchers, and there is lack of consensus on the impact it has on death anxiety. A study by Duff and Hong (1995) found that death anxiety was lower in communities with a high rate of attendance at religious services. The communities with the highest frequency of attendance of religious services scored significantly lower in death anxiety than communities with lower attendance. However, what is not clear from this study is whether attendance alone was a significant factor in determining level of death anxiety. Consideration should be given to how religious motivation and the strength of one's belief might predict the levels of death anxiety one may experience. Attendance may be seen as just 'going through the motions' without the intrinsic religious conviction and motivation. It is therefore important first to make the distinction between frequent attendance and intrinsic religious conviction, and then to determine the levels of death anxiety for each group. Those with an intrinsic religious conviction tend to believe in life after death. According to Rose and O'Sullivan (2002) a belief in life after death is therefore employed as a buffer against death anxiety. However, the assumption from this is rightly or wrongly based on the notion that life after death itself is rewarding enough to look forward to it. This view appears weak and limited as long as there is a lack of clear concrete evidence of what constitutes life after death.

Death anxiety and health care professionals

Understanding of the different perspectives of death anxiety and the possible sources and variables that can modify it all help in our quest to minimise its impact on health care professionals. It is obvious that not every health care professional will respond in the same way when exposed to death and dying experiences of adult patients. Each professional brings a unique perception of life, health, illness and death, suggesting that the impact of witnessing patients' death and dying episodes will be equally different. In addition to these individual differences, the nature and quality of social support received by these professionals from their managers and employing organisation also helps them remain resilient to the demands of caring for dying patients.

Man's futile attempt

A futile attempt to keep death anxiety under check (Neimeyer and Brunt, 1995), for both professionals and patients/families is to engage in ritualistic reassurances that are in themselves obviously false but mask the impulse to panic or run away from it all. Generally some people will often use euphemisms to hide or minimise death anxiety. This is also common amongst health professionals, particularly those caring for dying patients. This psychological indulgence in euphemisms is important for them as a way of 'buffering' or softening the impact of death anxiety. In other words, it makes discussion around death more palatable. Table 2.3 lists six common categories of euphemisms used in relation to someone who has died.

The role of euphemisms

People's tendency to use euphemisms as a defence against death anxiety is most likely to begin with their cultural and religious socialisation. For most people their dependence on parents and society as role models may have a lot

Table 2.3 Common euphemisms.

Journey euphemisms	Rest euphemisms	Loss euphemisms
The departed	Gone to eternal rest	No longer with us
Cross the great divide	Resting in peace	Will be sadly missed
Go to meet one's	Go to one's rest	Society has lost...
maker	Now in Heaven	The greatest
Go to the happy hunt-	Everlasting sleep	With fond memories
ing ground	Everlasting peace	Reported missing
Joining the angels		Unaccounted for
Joining one's ancestors		Off the record
A big send-off		
Reward euphemisms	**Joy euphemisms**	**End euphemisms**
No more suffering	Peaceful	The late...
No more pain	In the arms of the	No more
Freedom of the soul	father	Deceased
Relieved of suffering	United with God	Time or number was
Called to rest	In heaven	up
	In Paradise	Presumed dead
	Singing with the angels	Debt we all must pay
		Pull the plug

to do with the eventual in-authenticity and self deception inherent in euphemisms. Just like the fear of the possibility of having no further existence, euphemisms express a pervasive fear of the unknown, hence the six categories of euphemisms listed in Table 2.3 go some way to justifying this claim. Fear of the loss of a loved one and fear of the possibility of death bring about the pseudo-humbleness expressed through euphemisms. The practice of using euphemisms for death is likely to have originated with the magical belief that to speak the word 'death' was to invite death; where to 'draw Death's attention' is the ultimate bad fortune – a common theory holds that death is a taboo subject in most English-speaking cultures for precisely this reason. It may be said that one is not dying, but *fading quickly* because *the end is near*. People who have died are referred to as having *passed away* or *passed* or *departed*. *Deceased* is a euphemism for 'dead', and sometimes the *deceased* is said to have *gone to a better place*, but this is used primarily among the religious with a concept of Heaven. The media and in particular newspaper obituaries seem a rich vein for such death euphemisms.

To recap, euphemisms serve to soften the impact of death on a family, a people, a community and a society. Secondly, euphemisms encourage the portrayal of positive perception within a death, while focusing on the 'good' aspects of the person who has died. It seems that a time of death is a time to forget/ignore or temporarily suspend any 'bad' or negative aspects about the dead person. The question that remains unanswered is whether such practices are aimed at reducing the possibility of death anxiety among the bereaved and society at large. From a psychological perspective, once positive attributes about the deceased are portrayed, it is arguable that this gives the survivors a sense of purpose and a perception that death can have positive outcome (i.e. by highlighting the 'good' things). It can be argued that although such practices are inauthentic, they help people cope with the death before them.

Concluding thoughts

The concept of death remains elusive to understand and let alone define. There are numerous permutations of what constitutes death. This chapter has explored some of the different definitions from physiological to psychospiritual perspectives. The diversity of perspectives suggests that death and its characteristics are complex to harness. The way people view and relate to death will inevitably influence their response to their own impending death. The knowledge of one's possibility of being dead (a state of non-being or nothingness) often triggers different reactions, some of which are geared to prevent death or prolong life. On a psychological level, the contemplation of the possibility of one's death may result in emotional reactions, of which death anxiety is one of the most potent and common. For those who witness other people's death and dying experiences, there is an argument to suggest that this might also impact on perceptions of their own mortality. Witnessing someone else's death is common for health care professionals in general and palliative care nurses in particular. What needs understanding is the impact on the palliative care nurses, in relation to their own death anxiety and perception of their mortality.

Although this chapter explored the irrationality of fearing death, the reality remains that people continue to do so. The chapter has given possible explanations as to why this happens, but the indiscriminate nature and meaning of death provoke the most anxiety among human beings.

Death anxiety is an emotion which can be moderated by factors like age, religious beliefs and in some cases gender. Nurses working in palliative care are of varying ages, religious beliefs and gender. Nurses in palliative care settings are constantly being exposed to the death and dying experiences of their patients. Such exposure is likely to raise the awareness of their own death, and the consequences can be far-reaching on the quality of care they provide.

It is not yet clear whether high levels of death anxiety might lead nurses to become more susceptible to job-related stress as well and eventually the burnout syndrome. This seems an interesting area for future research study.

References

Abdel-Khalek, A. M. (2002) Why do we fear death? The construction and validation of the reasons for death fear scale. *Death Studies*, **26**, 669–80.

Appignanesi, R. (2006) *What Do Existentialists Believe?* Granta Books, London.

Becker, E. (1973) *The Denial of Death*. Free Press, New York.

Belsky, J. (1999) *The Psychology of Ageing*. Brookes Cole, New York.

Berman, A. L. and Hays, J. E. (1973) Relationship between death anxiety, belief in afterlife and locus of control. *Journal of Consulting and Clinical Psychology*, **41**(2), 318.

Duff, R. and Hong, L. (1995) Age density, religiosity and death anxiety in retirement communities. *Reviews of Religious Research*, **37**, 19–32.

Erickson, E. H. (1963) *Childhood and Society*. Norton, New York.

Erickson, E. H. (1982) *The Life Cycle Completed*. Norton, New York.

Feifel, H. (1959) *The Meaning of Death*. McGraw-Hill, New York.

Freud, S. (1953) *Thoughts for the Times on War and Death*. Hogarth Press, London.

Freud, S. (1961) *Beyond the Pleasure Principle*. Leverringht Publishing Company, New York.

Goebel, B. L. and Boeck, B. E. (1987) Ego integrity and fear of death: a comparison of institutionalised and independently living older adults. *Death Studies*, **11**, 193–204.

Greenberg, J., Koole, L. S. and Pyszczynski, T. (Eds.) (2004) *Handbook of Experimental Existential Psychology*. The Guildford Press, New York.

Heidegger, M. (1962) *Being and Time*. Blackwell Publishing, Oxford.

Hickson, J., Housely, W. F. and Boyle, C. (1988) The relationship of locus of control, age and sex to life satisfaction and death anxiety in older persons. *International Journal of Aging and Human Development*, **20**, 191–9.

Hinohara, S. (1948) *The Life of Dr W. Osler – a Pioneer in American Medicine*. Chuo Igakusha, Tokyo.

Honderich, T. (ed.) (2005) *The Oxford Companion to Philosophy*. Oxford University Press, Oxford.

Jaspers, K. (1951) *The Way to Wisdom*. Yale University Press, London.

Kamm, F. M. (1998) Why is death bad and worse than pre-natal non-existence? *Pacific Philosophical Quarterly*, **69**, 161–4.

Kastenbaum, R. J. (1986) *Death, Society, and Human Experience*. Charles E. Merrill, Columbus.

Kastenbaum, R. J. (2000) *The Psychology of Death*, 3rd edn. Springer, New York.

Kierkegaard, S. (1844) *The Concept of Dread*. Princeton Unversity Press, Princeton.

Kierkegaard, S. (1847) *Purity of Heart is to Will One Thing*. Harper & Row, New York.

Langford, I. H. (2002) An existential approach to risk perception. *Risk Analysis*, **22**(1), 101–20.

Langs, R. (1997) *Death Anxiety and Clinical Practice*. Kamac Books, London.

Langs, R. (2004) Death anxiety and the emotion-processing mind. *Psychoanalytic Psychology*, **21**(1), 31–53.

Lester, D. (1994) The Collett–Lester Fear of Death Scale. In: *Death Anxiety Handbook: Research, Instrumentation, and Application* (ed. R. A. Neimeyer). Taylor & Francis, Washington.

Lonetto, R. and Templer, D. I. (1986) *Death Anxiety*. Hampshire Publishing Corporation, Washington.

Lucretius (1951) *On the Nature of the Universe*. Penguin, London.

May, R. (1977) *The Meaning of Anxiety*, rev edn. Norton, New York.

McCarthy, J. (1980) *Death Anxiety: The Loss of Self*. Gardner Press, New York.

Nagel, T. (1970) Death. *Nous*, **4**, 73–80.

Neimeyer, R. A. (1994) *Death Anxiety Handbook: Research, Instrumentation, and Application*. Taylor & Francis, Washington.

Neimeyer, R. A. and Brunt, D. V. (1995) Death anxiety. In: *Dying; Facing the facts* (eds. H. Wass and R. A. Neimeyer). Taylor & Francis, Washington.

Nyatanga, B. (2005) Is fear of death itself a rational preoccupation? *International Journal of Palliative Nursing*, **11**(12), 643–5.

Nyatanga, B. and de Vocht, H. (2006) Towards a definition of death anxiety. *International Journal of Palliative Nursing*, **12**(9), 410–13.

Pallis, C. and Harley, D. H. (1996) *ABC of Brainstem Death*, 2nd edn. British Medical Journal, London.

Parfit, D. (1984) *Reasons and Persons*. Clarendon Press, Oxford.

Park, J. (2001) *An Existential Understanding of Death: a Phenomenology of Ontological Anxiety*, 4th edn. Available from: http://www.existentialbooks.com/ (Accessed on May 2005).

Parkes, C. M. (1978) Psychosocial transitions: a field for study. *Social Science and Medicine*, **5**, 101–14.

Quinn, P. K. and Reznikoff, M. (1985) The relationship between death anxiety and the subjective experience of time in the elderly. *International Journal of Aging and Human Development*, **21**, 197–209.

Rasmussen, C. A. and Brems, C. (1996) The relationship of death anxiety with age and psychosocial maturity. *The Journal of Psychology*, **130**, 141–4.

Rose, B. and O'Sullivan, M. J. (2002) Afterlife beliefs and death anxiety: an exploration of the relationship between afterlife expectations and fear of death in an undergraduate population. *Omega: Journal of Death and Dying*, **45**(3), 229–43.

Rosenbaum, S. E. (1989) The symmetry argument: Lucretius against the fear of death. *Philosophy and Phenomenological Research*, **1**(2).

Rotter, J. B., Seeman, M. and Liverant, S. (1962) Internal versus external control of reinforcements: A major variable in behavior theory. In: *Decisions, Values, and Groups*, Vol. 2 (ed. N. F. Washburne). Pergamon, London.

Sherman, D. W. (1997) Correlates of death anxiety in nurses who provide AIDS care. *Omega: Journal of Death & Dying*, **34**(2), 117–37.

Smieja, M., Kalaska, M. and Adamczyk, M. (2006) Scared to death or scared to love? Terror Management Theory and close relationship seeking. *European Journal of Social Psychology*, **36**, 279–96.

Stokes, P. (2006) *Philosophy. 100 Essential Thinkers*. Arcturus, London.

Templer, D. (1970) The construction and validation of a death anxiety scale. *Journal of General Psychology*, **82**, 165–77.

Thorson, J. A. and Powell, F. C. (1988) Elements of death anxiety and meanings of death. *Journal of Clinical Psychology*, **44**, 691–701.

Tillich, P. (1952) *The Courage to Be*. Yale University Press, New Haven.

Tomer, A. and Eliason, G. (1996) Toward a Comprehensive Model of Death Anxiety. *Death Studies*, **20**, 343–65.

Toscani, F., Cantoni, L., Di Mola, G., Mori, M., Santosuosso, A. and Tamburini, M. (1991) Death and dying: Perceptions and attitudes in Italy. *Palliative Medicine*, **5**, 334–343.

Weston, D. (1996) *Psychology. Mind, Brain & Culture*. John Wiley & Sons, New York.

Williams, K. (2005) *Why the Fear of Death Itself is Irrational*. Available from: http://www.near-death.com/experiences/articles007 (accessed 4 December 2005).

CHAPTER 3

A paradigm of death

Brian Nyatanga

It is impossible to imagine your own death, and whenever we attempt to do so, we can perceive that we are in fact still present as spectators (Freud, 1953)

Introduction

The major academic disciplines have tried to understand the nature of death by compartmentalising it in a way that is palatable for them. Psychology (Morgan, 1995) views death in terms of an end result of a process of suffering. Here the context of suffering relates to all the different dimensions that make up a person, and is not restricted only to the physical. Dying itself is characterised by suffering 'total' pain that encompasses the psycho-emotional, physical, social, spiritual, intellectual and legal (PEPSSIL) dimensions of the person. The experiences that people have in life contribute to pain, regret, fear of the unknown and guilt, and all this amounts to suffering. Sociology considers death as the final phase of performing the different roles such as being a mother, a sister, a wife and/or a daughter to someone. This often provokes emotional reactions from the dying person and those of significance. Inevitably, where there is an emotional reaction people need to be encouraged to *work through their grief*[1]. Philosophy (Frankl, 1963) views death as a bringing about of distinctive fears of non-existence, meaninglessness or extinction with no significance. Finally, religion views death as a Holy passage from this life to another eternal existence. To be guaranteed this eternal existence the indi-

---

1 This term comes from the psychodynamic arena, and is specifically Freudian. Freud's basic view was that grief needs to be confronted, to be 'worked through'. Freud saw detachment or withdrawal of libido from the lost object as essential before the grieving person can re-establish or re-invest the libidinal energy with another person(s). Therefore this process of 'Working Through' was seen as a prerequisite before the bereaved could move on into a new life. (See also Chapter 9.)

vidual should live his or her life according to the teachings of the Holy Spirit or relevant doctrine.

This philosophical position is fundamental in our attempt to understand why many people find it difficult to die and talk about death openly. This reluctance makes people conjure up different mental images of death, and hence death continues to be viewed as a taboo subject, particularly in Western societies. Aries (1974) claims that death is so frightful that people dare not utter its name. Since Aries' claim, things have changed, in that now there is an enormous volume of writing on the topic of death. However, the paradox is whether people, exposed to such voluminous writings, go on to talk about their *own* death. While death is the only certainty in life (Field and James, 1993) and there is one death per person, it continues to be handled 'badly'. I do not believe that death is the problem, but that the actual process of dying is. Considering all the care and resources available, dying remains a lonely passage in that no individual can live through the experience of terminality for another (Feifel, 1977). As well as the physical process, dying has psycho-social, philosophical and spiritual passages and the nature of those passages may be influenced by others. For example, in a social passage, what happens to the dying person is greatly affected by other people, who form part of his or her social world. Some of you may well remember the patient who 'puts off' dying until his son arrives from abroad or a grandchild is born. Is there a real influence or power from the son/grandchild or is this mere physiological coincidence? On the other hand, could it be in the patient's power to control his own destiny in such a precise manner?

The knowledge or realisation that one is dying induces anxiety and fear. Such death fear will be discussed later in this chapter. Dying is often viewed as synonymous with pain and suffering. This suffering applies both to the person who is dying and to those close to him. Dying itself as a process can be avoided, and hence more and more people are asking for ways of avoiding or missing out part of their passage or transition when their own death is imminent. It is clear that you and I will die one day, but it is not that clear that dying will be part of our life. For example, those who suffer a myocardial infarction (MI) or fatal road traffic accident (RTA) like Diana, Princess of Wales and Dodi Al-Fayed, avoid the prolonged process (passage) of dying. This, however, would not be everyone's chosen way of avoiding the process of dying; people are now asking for more humane or controlled ways of achieving death. Proponents of euthanasia, physician-assisted suicide and mercy killing are campaigning for the omission or avoidance of this passage, presumably for those who are suffering. They all point out the degree of suffering experienced by the dying person. By ending the suffering and pain they also stop the process of dying. What this argument may be suggesting is that without the suffering, people would tolerate dying. This is worth thinking hard about, particularly for those of us working in palliative care, where death and dying are a common phenomenon. A fundamental point to remember about dying is that it often affects one's overall quality of life. Here quality of life should be seen as unique to the individual, but may be often determined by others (like in a social passage), without finding out whether the individual him- or herself really wants as quality of life. What needs considering is this emphasis on quality of life when one has a terminal illness, as if this never existed in his life before the diagnosis. The truth is that everybody has his or her own quality of life with or without a terminal illness, and this can be traced from birth to adulthood on a continuum. What I see as the problem with dying is that even those who had not valued the quality of their life when they were well and healthy are somewhat encouraged and persuaded to believe in and adopt a better or different quality of life. This is often set by the institution for the dying such as hospices. The paradox is whether the resultant quality of life is for the patient or perhaps those in charge of the patient's day-to-day care.

When dying is avoided through MI or RTA, there is shock and disbelief in those left behind, although on the other hand it may be seen as a blessing. For those who see it as a blessing, you could argue that they are trying to get rid of dying altogether as a precursor to death. Dying itself, as mentioned earlier, is characterised by suffering 'total' pain that encompasses the PEPSSIL dimensions of the person. This would hold true for the dying person and significant others who will be left behind. The realisation that dying causes enormous suffering forms the basis of the hospice philosophy and palliative care provision. Although the concept of a 'good' death seems popular in palliative care, Neuberger (1994) argues that this can be alien to other cultural groups such as the Jewish. It is worth exploring the notion of a good death using Bayliss's (1996) three categories. According to Bayliss, it is possible to have a medically 'good' death, which is characteristic of pain and other distressing symptoms being well controlled. It is also possible to have a naturally 'good' death such as in old age. Here death is expected and is caused by natural ageing process. The third category is seen as a religious or culturally 'good' death, where enough warning is given in order to carry out certain rituals before death occurs. This brief review of a 'good' death highlights the diversity of this notion. What then is important is to understand individual ways of viewing dying and hence their own individual paradigm of death, and help them to achieve it; for example, what is considered a 'good' medical death might be perceived as 'bad' if it contravened cultural imperatives.

People tend to live their dying in different ways (Morgan, 1995). These ways are arguably dependent on three main aspects:

- The way people think about dying (*Cognitive* dimension)
- The way people feel about dying (*Affective* dimension)
- What people do when faced with dying (*Behavioural* dimension)

The behavioural component as a response is, arguably, largely influenced by the other two (cognitive and affective). In other words, behaviour tends to be the observable physical manifestation of the cognitive and affective processes as people interact with and react to their dying. Some of these reactions are well documented in the staged model of dying by Kubler-Ross (1970) and how to achieve an appropriate death (Weisman, 1972). If this analogy is acceptable it follows then that people whose cognitive and or affective dimensions are not functioning, wholly or partially, would lack an observable congruent behaviour in response to their dying or that of significant others. It is worth taking a deep look at your own views at this point. For example, if you did not think of or feel anything towards your dying sister, your behaviour towards her dying would, most likely, not affect your PEPSSIL dimensions, and hence it would be a non-specific reaction. This non-specificity is a mere interpretation of that behaviour given the expected norms of your group of people or society at large. There may not be a clear-cut explanation of this non-specificity because of the differences in individuals. It is always worth thinking of cultural variations and their kaleidoscopic nature (Devito, 1992; Nyatanga, 1997).

It would not suffice to talk about a paradigm of dying without placing emphasis on the social and cultural environments that impinge on the dying process of each individual. People's thought processes and feelings are greatly influenced and learned through such environments. In addition, there is a possible paradigm shift in response to changes in cultures or their key features. Cultures may change due to exposure to other cultures, the media, peer influence or direct contacts. Devito (1992) refers to such changes as acculturation. What may be fascinating in this process is that, while these changes take place, O'Neill (1995) argues that the rituals and practices at birth and marriage and during dying may not change.

A death system

Kastenbaum and Aisenberg (1972) maintain that a death system is characterised by two main factors: factual and theoretical. Factual characteristics would include things like how exposed to death and dying one is. The expected longevity of one's life may influence reactions to dying. For example, the current life expectancy of men in the UK is shorter than that of women.

The second aspect, theoretical factors, examines the way in which individuals perceive themselves as having control over the forces of nature, and also of an individual's meaning of being a person.

Experience as a factual determinant of death

The experience that an individual has about dying may influence greatly his understanding and awareness of death. The awareness levels will be discussed later on in this chapter. Experiences will be varied and the point to consider is whether such a diversity may have different influences on the individual. Consider an individual who experiences death in the course of his duty of working in a hospital, and another individual whose experience was the death of a close loved one. The other extreme of the argument is that an individual with no experience of death may have a limited or wholly intellectual/abstract attitude toward death. It is now claimed that people who have had near-death experiences change their attitude toward death (Greyson, 1992). It can be argued that a hospital staff member may be more aware of the nature of dying than a brewer. But more professional experience may not mean personal experience

Another factor to consider is how long people live (life expectancy). For some young people, raised in a family that tends to live as long as 70+ years old, it is possible that their first personal or close encounter with dying will be in their mid-thirties. Arguably their death system will be shaped differently from those of people who grow up in war-torn zones of the world, and also where people die from starvation, such as in Ethiopia, Rwanda and Bosnia. Those who die will be both young as well as old. Life expectancy has been changing over the years. Lerner (1970) claims that at the beginning of the 20th century life expectancy was not more than 40 years. Obviously such figures reflect an average, since some people would have lived to over 70 years, while others died as young as five. Lerner (1970) claims that one other reason for the low life expectancy was that many women died in childbirth.

Control of nature

The way individuals view the world that they live in and the extent of their perceived control of nature may shape their death system. There are forces of nature that play a part in our perception of death. One argument is that those who perceive themselves as having control over the forces of nature have a different view of death from those who see the forces of nature as having control. Perhaps by considering the following views, you may want to decide for yourself your own perception of and attitude to death. One view is that nature is actually there to be controlled and used by human beings. Such a view may encourage human beings to determine their own destiny and control their dying. You could possibly think of examples for this; and in some cases nature is used to perpetuate the enjoyment of human beings. The other view is that nature is there to be respected and protected. The emphasis here is that human beings are already an integral part of nature. With such partnership the main aim is to bring the best out of each other. It is about nurturing nature in order for it to protect the individual. Those holding such a view may 'allow' nature to influence their death and hence believe in fatalism.

On being a person

The notion of being a person forms the other theoretical factor (Kastenbaum and Aisenberg, 1972) that shapes a death system. In the field of palliative care, the central tenet of care is based on treating the patient as a person. Each person is unique, presenting with specific needs and characteristics. The question that needs exploring is what it is to be a person. A holistic approach to care suggests that a person is a complex whole with mental, social and emotional as well as physical characteristics. Reed and Ground (1997) argue that this is often called into question when one of them (mental or physical characteristics) is not functional for whatever reason. Of the two characteristics, the mental ability tends to influence or have more significance and dominance over the physical, even in pain perception, despite the evidence from the physical phenomenology of living. In other words, the mental aspect of the person is the more fundamental of the two. Reed and Ground give examples of mindless bodies such as algae and the vegetable kingdom, where there is life but which could not be classified as a person. This poses dilemmas for carers in palliative care and other related settings, where the minds of patients may be impaired as a result of their illness or their medication. It would be myopic to think of a person in terms of his or her mental activities, as this may lead to ill treatment of patients as living objects. In addition to this philosophical perspective, the emphasis of being a person can be seen from cultural and societal variations. According to Morgan (1995) Western cultures place emphasis on the uniqueness of the person and his or her rights. Other cultures emphasise that a person is part of a whole, that is, focusing on a group or species in which he or she is a part. Cultural orientations lead the person to hold different views about death. There is another extreme where the person is perceived as having no meaning at all, therefore calling into question the whole notion of existence of that person. Where a person is viewed as a whole, the social context of death comes into sharper focus (Morgan, 1995). This focus may determine the person's death system and consequently shape attitudes toward death. To determine a person's death system, there is a need to understand the basis of the attitude, fear and expectations about death. Such attributes are often an indication of the person's awareness of impending death as well as his or her individuality. It may be useful at this point to explore well-known contexts of awareness in order to explain the points made above.

Although many authors have studied death and dying (Kubler-Ross (1970) stages the process in psycho-social dimensions, Shneidman (1977) considers it as a set of responses to challenges and Weisman (1978) sees it as goal-orientated, aiming to achieve an appropriate death), the work of Glaser and Strauss (1965) on contexts of awareness will form the basis of the exploration.

Contexts of awareness

The contexts of awareness offer a sociological perspective on dying. Glaser and Strauss (1965) base their study on observing dying people and their patterns of communication. Glaser and Strauss claim that dying people go through four phases of awareness of their impending death, namely closed awareness (CA), suspected awareness (SA), mutual pretence (MP) and open awareness (OA).

In *closed awareness* the dying person is in 'total darkness' about his or her impending death. The relatives and health care professionals are the only ones who know and tend to engage in a secret pact of keeping this information from the dying person. There are possible reasons for this behaviour, including families being very protective towards the dying person, or health care professionals being reluctant to say death was imminent. It is also possible that the dying person may not be familiar with the symptoms of impending death (Glaser and Strauss, 1965).

However, the notion of closed awareness itself is confusing or contradictory in that the two terms, *closed* and *awareness* suggest two parallels, or different states of being. If one is aware, the interpretation is that there is some degree of knowing, albeit it is minimal. To be closed, on the other hand, would suggest total darkness, no awareness at all, no clue, complete ignorance as to what is happening. Perhaps less contradictory terms may be *total darkness* or *unawareness*.

Suspected awareness is a state of being when the dying person suspects his or her poor prognosis. What he or she may be looking for is either validation or disapproval of these suspicions by family or health care professionals. It would not be surprising to find that most dying people would hope for disapproval, perhaps a reflection of the death-denying attitude of the society we live in. The suspicion is often aroused by changes in the attitudes and behaviours of family and others, including treatment regimens. Treatment may change from curative to palliative, therefore focusing on the quality of life. The worsening condition is often characterised by weight loss, which is probably the single most obvious sign to raise suspicion.

Mutual pretence is psychologically the most challenging period for health care professionals. Glaser and Strauss (1965) claim that, at this point, the dying person, family and carers are aware of the poor prognosis but choose, by some kind of subconscious agreement, not to talk about the impending death. Glaser and Strauss see this as a game of pretending, where all the 'players' continually have a mutual conspiracy not to admit openly the reality of the illness. There are many possible reasons for this behaviour, including emotional distancing from the dying person by the health care professionals. The relatives I encountered in clinical practice came over as being protective of their loved one. They felt that discussing the poor prognosis openly would result in the dying person 'giving up' the fight. On the other hand the dying person often felt that the fact that he was dying was distressing enough for the family, without the added hurt and worry of talking openly about it. Therefore, in most cases silence on the matter was seen as a better option. While there may be a sound rationale for this, what we should ask ourselves is whether this may mean missed opportunities to say 'goodbye' or 'I am sorry'. It may exist because health care professionals protect themselves by not 'reading' the signals that indicate that people want to talk. While it may be argued that mutual pretence is necessary in order to retain a modicum of emotional stability, this may also prevent dialogue about practical arrangements such as wills, insurance and property.

Open awareness is the fourth phase which exists when the dying person, family and health care professionals acknowledge and talk openly with the dying person. It is here that essential facts are discussed openly amongst the three parties. The practical arrangements or rearrangements are made; for example, writing a new will or changing an existing one. The dying person may be preparing for death, practically, but nobody will ever know what is going on in the person's subconscious mind. Although the behaviour in this phase suggests acceptance of the reality of their death (at a conscious level) they may remain unconsciously terrified of its occurrence (Firestone, 1994). Although it may seem superfluous to carers, accepting this realisation may bring fear to patients from the knowledge of what is really happening or imminent. Constant interaction is needed in order to offer assurances, to provide answers to questions about care options and the effects of medication, to involve children, and to provide religious reaffirmation. Health care professionals may find it difficult working in open awareness, as the dying person may request full information about their condition and illness.

Death fear

There is an element of fear attached to every dying, even though outwardly people may be exhibiting behaviours that suggest acceptance of the reality. One argument is that the more aware of dying people become the more terrified they are, and this intensifies the fear of death.

There are many terms that have been used to refer to death fear, such as death concern, death threat and death anxiety (Neimeyer, 1994) and these have been used interchangeably in the literature. What needs discussing is whether there is any difference between these terms. For the purposes of this argument, only death fear and death anxiety will be discussed. These two terms also seem to be the most used or referred to in the available literature. According to Neimeyer and Brunt (1995, p. 52), establishing a difference between death fear and death anxiety has always been supported by those working psychodynamically, who link the experience of anxiety with the expression of unconscious conflict. However, since the psychodynamic approach has lost considerable momentum lately (Neimeyer and Brunt, 1995), this has led to the theoretical basis for distinction between fear and anxiety becoming less attractive. When used in practical terms (that is, with tools or equipment measuring apprehension about death), fear and anxiety are equivalent, assuming consistency and suitability are ensured. It has to be noted that the measurement tools are themselves subject to considerable debate, because most scales are thought to be unreliable.

The death fear that will be discussed here is what Tomer (1994) refers to as the anticipation of the state in which one is dead. This will also depend on what perspective one employs to try to make sense of death. For this chapter, only the perspectives of psychology and philosophy will form the bulk of the discussion. Before turning to these, however, we will take a brief look at gender differences relating to death fear.

Death fear and gender difference

It is thought that a difference does exist in death fear between males and females. However, the nature of the difference is still poorly understood (Neimeyer, 1990). Several studies that have been carried out. Pollack (1979) showed that women are more prone to reveal their death fear than men. The discrepancy can be seen from women's greater ability or readiness to reveal openly their feelings than men. While men may not readily admit or reveal their feelings, it should not be misconstrued as a lack of death fear. Men tend not to show their emotions easily; generally this is a Western view, but it is more specifically a Eurocentric view. Some studies have found no differences at all between the sexes (Stillion, 1985). What is of interest is that the factors that induce death fear in both males and females are similar. Leming and Dickinson (1994) identified nine such factors based on the impending death of self and the death of others. The box overleaf is an outline of the factors, which are also intertwined and tend to potentiate one another.

Factors that induce death fear in both males and females

- Dependency
- Pain in dying process
- Leaving loved ones
- Indignity of the dying process
- Isolation
- Separation
- Rejection
- Afterlife concerns
- Fate of the body

The finality of death

On the other hand there are exceptions to the above, in that not everyone will experience death fear. Leming and Dickinson (1994) claim that when B. F. Skinner[2] was dying (at 86 years old) he talked openly about his knowledge of his impending death. He said he was not worried or anxious, as he always knew that he was going to die. There seems to be a degree of acceptance of the reality of death in this case, and this may also be based on the fact that Skinner had, in his own way, achieved most if not all that he wanted. His work was successful and being used by academics and students, influencing their way of thinking and behaviour.

Philosophical perspectives

The knowledge that we are unable to continue as a 'being' evokes a state of fear in us. Death itself becomes the ultimate threat to our existence, and realisation of such a threat brings about fear or anxiety. Using Heidegger's postulates, the realisation of our impending non-existence is a precondition for understanding our life and eventually a precursor to freeing ourselves from fear (Heidegger, 1962). This is supposedly dependent on our actual construction of death in our

---

2 Skinner (1904–1990) was a prominent psychologist who espoused theories on programmed learning and behaviour modification using rats and pigeons.

minds. For death to be viewed as freedom, its meaning must be established and should encompass it as being more than a threat to existence.

The other way of looking at death fear is to use Sartre's view, which is to see death as actually getting in the way of a person's potential and capabilities (Sartre, 1966). Death has the ability to reduce a person to a state of nothingness. Nothingness is like looking through a mirror of our meaninglessness in terms of our existence. Using Sartre's view, it can be argued that because people are constantly thinking of their death, there is a propensity to higher levels of death fear. Death, in essence, reminds us of our past, or that which has been. If for example a person's life is not complete (complete being used in the subjective dimension), death may provoke a lot more fear or anxiety than in someone who has fulfilled his or her ambitions and other expectations, for example B. F. Skinner, as discussed above. Where life is not complete, death is seen as an unwelcome, as well as an untimely interruption of one's life. This bears resemblance to the psychological perspective of self-actualisation (personological) theories such as that of Maslow (1968). According to these theories, self-actualising individuals tend to have a higher acceptance of themselves, and hence less fear of any unfinished accomplishments and consequently have a lower death fear. Self-actualisation may be a way of reinforcing a person's self-worth. Self-worth is about bringing out the real self by realising or achieving what a person really wishes to be. What one wishes to be is arguably the acquired spiritual dimension of that person.

Psychological perspectives

Death fear can be explained by exploring theories that search for meaning (Frankl, 1963). The realisation that death is imminent 'forcibly' makes the person review his perception, outlook, future plans and expectations in an attempt to rediscover a new sense of purpose in his life. In order to accomplish this, it becomes crucially imperative that the person has an appreciation of his relationship with the past. Frankl (1963, p. 122) wrote 'In the past, nothing is irrecoverably lost but everything irrevocably stored'. This is a clear demonstration that the past is the only certainty of the person's being, and true meaning can therefore be derived from it. Another way of looking at this is to see life as full of potentialities that are in search of actualisation. Once actualised, they are rendered realities immediately, stored, 'sealed' and delivered into the past (Frankl, 1963).

Another different perspective used to look at death fear is that of constructs (Kelly, 1955), where a person tends to construe what is happening at present in order to predict similar events happening in the future.

Constructs can be either core or peripheral. Core constructs are those belief systems deeply held by the individual, and to change these would require major and radical reviews of the belief system and entire outlook (Tomer, 1994). Peripheral ones are loosely held and can be easily changed depending on the situation. It follows that death threatens the core constructs, therefore causing radical changes to a person's outlook. When this happens it will induce high levels of death fear. What tends to happen is that the person finds it difficult to make sense of death, and Tomer (1994) claims that any event that cannot be subsumed often causes fear. For religious people, this fear may be to do with how their life on this earth will be judged in order to make the 'transition' to eternity. Eternity is the ultimate goal for religious people and the 'entry passport' depends on whether life on earth was lived according to set commandments.

For other psychological theories to explain death fear, the reader is referred to Neimeyer's (1994) handbook on death anxiety.

Concluding thoughts

It is evident from the content of this chapter that there are many facets influencing a person's paradigm of death. The most prominent influences are rooted in past experiences with death itself, either physically or conceptually. Some of the experiences may have involved very close people or have been encountered during a course of duty, and therefore the impact may be different. Cultural and societal expectations tend to play a major role in shaping a person's paradigm. Such a paradigm is not innate but rather learned from individual families, peers, and social and cultural environments. Holding such a paradigm would enable the individuals to afford symbolic significance to human mortality (Kastenbaum and Aisenberg, 1972); see also Chapter 8 on the role of funerals. In addition to individuals holding their own paradigm, it is also obvious that different practice settings have their own perceptions of a paradigm of death. Arguably the hospital wards (medical, surgical, paediatric, A&E or orthopaedic) have their own way of caring for a dying patient and therefore affording that patient a way of dying (hence of paradigm of death). Hospice settings are often credited with good practice because of the way in which they afford the patient a way of dying that is unique to that patient. It can be argued that hospices try to follow as closely as possible a paradigm of death as preferred by the patient. Nursing homes care for the dying patients and the way of dying may be different from that found in hospitals and hospices. One argument for the different paradigms of death is the influence of the philosophy of care applied by each practice setting. What you may need to explore is why there are these different philosophies in caring for the dying patient in the various practice settings discussed above. It is well known that most people prefer to die at home, and this suggests that the home setting often affords them a paradigm of death in a homely environment.

The other factor to consider is the availability of resources, both human and equipment (material), as these also influence a patient's way of dying.

I have argued that death may not be the problem but that the actual process of dying is, since there is evidence from pro-euthanasia campaigners of a wish or desire to avoid this process. The realisation that death is imminent, together with the meaning attached to it, often leads to a state of fear or anxiety. This chapter has used some philosophical as well as psycho-social theories to explain the possible causes of death fear. It is my belief that when there is increased understanding of what causes death fear for each dying person, better care will follow and help to make dying easier.

In our quest to understand why it is so difficult to die, the next chapter will explore the role of medicine and nursing in death and dying. The medicalisation of death will be analysed to see whether it exacerbates or ameliorates dying and for whom. This chapter will also be the start of Part 2 of the book, where I consider death as the 'business' of others. The argument being advanced in Part 2 is about how dying, which used to be a quiet family affair, has been literally taken over by others: that is professionals and business-orientated people.

References

Aries, P. (1974) *Western Attitudes toward Death. From the Middle Ages to the Present.* Marion Boyars, New York.

Bayliss, V. J. (1996) *Understanding Loss and Grief.* National Extension College, Cambridge.

Devito, J. (1992) *The Interpersonal Communication Book*, 6th edn. HarperCollins, New York.

Feifel, H. (1977) *New Meanings of Death.* McGraw-Hill, New York.

Field, D. and James, N. (1993) Where and how people die. In: *The Future of Palliative Care* (ed. D. Clarke). Open University Press, Buckingham.

Firestone, R. W. (1994) Psychological defences against death anxiety. In: *Death Anxiety Handbook: Research, Instrumentation and Application* (ed. R. A. Neimeyer). Taylor & Francis, Washington.

Frankl, V. E. (1963) *Man's Search for Meaning.* Beacon Press, Boston.

Freud, S. (1953) *Thoughts for the Times on War and Death.* Hogarth Press, London.

Glaser, B. G. and Strauss, A. L. (1965) *Awareness of Dying.* Aldine, Chicago.

Greyson B. (1992) Reduced death threat in near-death experiences. *Death Studies,* **16**, 523–36.

Heidegger, M. (1962) *Being and Time.* SCM Press, London.

Kastenbaum, R. and Aisenberg, R. (1972) *The Psychology of Death.* Springer, New York.

Kelly, G. (1955) *A Theory of Personality – the Psychology of Personal Constructs.* Norton, New York.

Kubler-Ross, E. (1970) *On Death and Dying.* Tavistock, London.

Leming, M. R. and Dickinson, G. E. (1994) *Understanding Dying, Death and Bereavement*, 3rd edn. Harcourt Brace, New York.

Lerner, M. (1970) When, why and where people die. In: *The Dying Patient* (eds. O. G. Brim, H. E. Freeman, S. Levine and N. A. Scotch). Russell Sage, New York.

Maslow, A. (1968) *Toward a Psychology of Being*, 2nd edn. Van Nostrand Reinhold, New York.

Morgan, J. D. (1995) Living our dying and our grieving: historical and cultural attitudes. In: *Dying: Facing the Facts* (eds. H. Wass and R. A. Neimeyer). Taylor & Francis, Washington.

Neimeyer, R. (1994) *Death Anxiety Handbook: Research, Instrumentation and Application.* Taylor & Francis, Washington.

Neimeyer, R. A. and Brunt, D. V. (1995) Death anxiety. In: *Dying; Facing the facts* (eds. H. Wass and R. A. Neimeyer). Taylor & Francis, Washington.

Neuberger, J. (1994) *Caring for People of Different Faiths.* Wolfe, London.

Nyatanga, B. (1997) Cultural issues in palliative care. *International Journal of Palliative Nursing*, **3**(4), 203–8.

O'Neill A. (1995) Cultural issues in palliative care. *European Journal of Palliative Care*, **2**(3), 127–31.

Pollack, J. M. (1979) Correlates of death anxiety: a review of empirical studies. *Omega*, **10**, 97–121.

Reed, J. and Ground, I. (1997) *Philosophy for Nursing.* Arnold, London.

Sartre, J.-P. (1966) *Being and Nothingness: An Essay on Phenomenological Ontology.* Citadel Press, New York.

Shneidman, E. S. (1977) Aspects of the dying process. *Psychiatric Annals*, **8**, 25–40.

Stillion, J. M. (1985) *Death and the Sexes.* McGraw-Hill, Washington.

Tomer, A. (1994) Death anxiety in adult life: theoretical perspectives. In: *Death Anxiety Handbook: Research, Instrumentation and Application* (ed. R. A. Neimeyer). Taylor & Francis, Washington.

Weisman, A. D. (1972) *On Dying and Denying: a Psychiatric Study of Terminality.* Behavioural Publications, New York.

Weisman, A. (1978) An appropriate death. In: *Death and Dying: Challenge and Change* (eds. R. Fulton, E. Markusen, G. Owen and J. L. Scheiber). Addison-Wesley, Reading MA.

Death as a business of others

CHAPTER 4

An overview of the medicalisation of death, and the part played by palliative medicine

Part 1: The background and benefits of medicine in the care of the dying

Craig Gannon

Introduction

There is an increasing array of medical interventions available to people with advanced illnesses. And it is rarely disputed that there is now a far greater medical presence within the care of the dying. However, it is unclear whether this increase represents progress or failure. Attempts to provide a balanced overview of the medicalisation of death can prove surprisingly difficult; the conflicting views within the literature appear revealing. As is often the case, the issue is not best defined by focusing on such extreme stances.

Firstly, the relevant terminology is frequently applied inconsistently. Secondly, the intention and components of medical care offered to dying patients are poorly understood and often misrepresented. And thirdly, the emotive nature of discussions pertaining to death inevitably evokes strong individual or historical opinions, which can cloud the issue further. These circumstances conspire to leave commonly voiced beliefs being ill informed, yet held with conviction. The resulting debate – is medicine a 'force for good' or 'major threat to health'? – appears unhelpful (Moynihan and Smith, 2002). Clinical and personal prejudices make these generalisations around extremes as common among health care professionals as they are in the general public. The real question we need to answer is 'how much medical input is right?'. Sadly, this 'how much...?' question is less provocative and consequently it rarely has a high profile within medicalisation debates.

Any meaningful review on the relative value of adding medical input into the care of the dying requires an objective perspective. This demands a shared understanding of the terminology, along with sufficient awareness of the remit and range of available health care interventions, in particular from palliative care services. Palliative care can play a prominent part in patients' care in the later stages of incurable illnesses, even when 'dying'. Reviewing the benefits and harms from current health care provision should better clarify the driving forces behind the witnessed increases in medical input delivered to dying patients, either the expectations and/or the desires of society, individual patients, and/or medicine.

The limitations of available definitions

'Medicalisation' is a relatively recent term, and, in spite of increasing usage, it remains a broad and imprecise concept. Over the last 5–10 years, dictionaries have increasingly defined 'medicalised' as: 'to view or treat as a medical concern, problem, or disorder' (dictionary.com, 2006). In the medical literature, the term *medicalisation* has been defined as 'the process of defining an increasing number of life problems as medical problems' and particularly applied to birth, sexuality, aging, unhappiness and death (Moynihan and Smith, 2002). The term appears necessary to reflect the rapidly increasing medical interventions and expenditure within modern medicine.

Moreover, while definitions of *medicalisation* appear descriptive and not judgemental, the term still carries a consistently negative impact targeted against health care (Clark, 2002). The very terminology conveys condemning overtones of the imposition of medicine on society and thus, *over*medicalisation. Indeed some see "medicalisation" as the unwinnable battle against death, pain, and sickness perpetrated by doctors potentially eroding our (society's) ability to cope with reality (Moynihan and Smith, 2002). Indeed research has confirmed that societies that spend more on health care are more likely to regard themselves as sick.

Of all the potential areas, 'the medicalisation of death' is particularly open to different interpretations. Literally, 'the medicalisation of death' could appear to mean the practice of medicine at the moment life is lost. Clearly this interpretation appears unhelpfully limited. Alternatively, the phrase might apply more broadly to any intervention intended to improve the well-being of dying patients and their families. Thus 'the medicalisation of death' can cross several dimensions.

- **Perceptions**: is 'the medicalisation of death' a reflection of death-denying attitudes, beliefs or behaviours within patients, health care professionals and/or society? Are doctors the perpetrators or victims in this shifting of opinion (Moynihan and Smith, 2002)?
- **Scope**: if 'the medicalisation of death' is meant to reflect the 'dying' process (rather than just the moment of death), does 'dying' carry the clinical meaning (a patient's final hours, days or short weeks) or the less specific meaning used in common parlance (i.e. the later stages of incurable illnesses). Moreover, could the phrase equally apply to any stage of a life-threatening illness (even from diagnosis, possibly many months or years) and/or extend into the care of the bereaved?
- **Health care professional presence**: is 'the medicalisation of death' merely the input from doctors during a terminal illness? Is it absolute, or can medical input at certain times (e.g. if a terminally ill patient is acutely unwell) still be 'allowed' without becoming labelled 'medicalisation'? And does this term only refer to doctors, or does it extend to include other conventional health care professionals? Nurses have been asked to combat the medicalisation caused by doctors, while acknowledging nurses can also contribute to medicalisation (Hall, 2003). Equally does 'medicalisation' apply to complementary therapists? If it does not, as complementary therapy will share many of the same drawbacks as medicine, why not?
- **Therapeutics**: is 'the medicalisation of death' limited to the use of prescribed medicines towards the end of life, possibly excluding non-drug manoeuvres, even if directed by doctors? And would medicalisation not include self-medicating with over-the-counter medicines or even sophisticated self-directed dietary manoeuvres, despite sharing all the same therapeutic problems, such as unpleasant side-effects and the burden of compliance?
- **Autonomy**: is 'the medicalisation of death' a reflection of individuals' perceived increasing handing over of control to health care professionals as death approaches, but not the handing over of similar interventions to possibly less well-placed family carers? Does any reliance on medicine automatically represent medicalisation, even if it appears to be empowering the patient, faced otherwise with simply acquiescing to a greater loss of autonomy caused by their disease?
- **Pathology**: does 'the medicalisation of death' restrict itself to patients dying from chronic progressive illness, or does the term include all causes of death equally, from relatively sudden deaths (e.g. failed attempts to save a road traffic accident victim) to dying of 'natural causes' in old age?

The 'medicalisation of death' was first used in health care literature in the late 1970s to describe the secular and institutionalised attitudes to death of 'modern' Western society, with the accompanying loss of traditional coping mechanisms (Bevan, 1998). At that time, Ivan Illich (1990) suggested that modern medicine had 'brought the epoch of the natural death to an end' (Clark, 2002). What we understand today by a 'natural death' and whether it should be missed as strongly as implied is unclear. A major focus for concern on the medicalisation of death stemmed from medical practice in the 1970s. Personal views disagree as to the lesser or greater need for concern now. It has been implied that this previous need for concern is increasingly outdated, with biomedical aspirations peaking in the 1960s (Hoy, 1999) or that those concerns from the 1970s were just the start: 'the biomedical model indisputably is getting out of hand' (Hall, 2003). Potentially this divergence reflects firstly a United Kingdom (UK) palliative care perspective of late-stage illness, contrasting with (secondly) an American oncological perspective of early-stage disease. This reveals the heterogeneous populations and widely contrasting treatment options potentially covered by 'the medicalisation of death'.

As a concept, 'the medicalisation of death' invites unhelpful generalisations around the wisdom of health care's involvement in the care of the dying. As some patients with life-threatening illnesses undoubtedly need medical interventions, it is naïve to polarise the value of medical input into 'all good' or 'all bad'. As every case is unique, the objectives, the methods, and the level of medical contact required will differ vastly for each patient and at differing times of their illness. Once this intricacy is realised, any umbrella term that attempts to cover all health care interventions for dying patients as one appears flawed. Similarly, the differing medical specialities and other health care professional actions cannot be grouped as if homogeneous, even for the convenience of criticism. To be equitable, any discussion of 'the medicalisation of death' requires an acknowledgement of the complexity of possible health care input that may be judged appropriate or inappropriate. Generalisations can never be made safely as to the wisdom of health care's involvement in the care of the dying.

Subsequently 'the medicalisation of death' has been used inconsistently, rarely as originally intended and often employed to deliver an air of authority to surprisingly divergent points of view. The spectrum of scenarios covered suggests that the phrase applies equally to non-medical as well as medical activity and can range from initiating cardiopulmonary resuscitation (CPR) to merely the presence of any health care workers at any stage of a terminal illness or sudden death. Paradoxically, euthanasia, arguably a truly medicalised death, has been suggested as an antidote to the medicalisation of death.

The remit of medicine

Outside of palliative care, medicine can appear to be focused on pursuing increasingly technical and ambitious interventions. While the science of medicine is rapidly advancing, the less tangible art of caring has not necessarily been abandoned. It is worth highlighting that medical practice is not, and never has been, restricted to curing disease as traditionally described. The medical mandate is dual, not only to preserve life, but also to relieve suffering. These *two* components are obligatory and fundamental to good practice. Thus once a disease has progressed beyond life-prolonging treatment, the medical remit becomes solely to relieve any suffering as defined by the individual patient. This professional remit reassuringly shapes an appropriate medical practice for dying patients. Medical investigations may be intended to provide invaluable prognostic information rather than direct heroic treatments and the majority of therapeutic inventions are likely to be non-pharmacological. Regardless, there is little objection to the reduction of pain or other distressing symptoms via medical means.

Medical practice is compelled by a basic framework for respecting the dignity of human life that remains singularly relevant in its application to the care of dying patients (Latimer, 1991; Stanley, 1992; Beauchamp and Childress, 1994). Four cardinal principles are described. When considered together they can be used as an approach to most bioethical situations:

- **Beneficence**: to do good, i.e. relieve suffering and enhance quality of life
- **Non-maleficence**: to do no harm, i.e. do not incur unnecessary tests or therapies/adverse effects
- **Patient autonomy**: to respect patients and their choices
- **Justice**: to fairly allocate resources to allow equally high-quality care to all in need

Thus medicine, though always respecting and striving to preserve life, when caring for dying patients is equally obligated to accept the inevitability of the patients' death (and discontinue any futile treatments), to facilitate patients' wishes to discontinue or not start any available treatments (or start/continue as appropriate), and to maintain patients' comfort and well being. This cements sound medical practice that should dispel the blanket negative responses that assume a harmful intrusion by medicine in the care of the dying. However, there are described limitations to these ethical principles: in the potential for different weighting of each factor; the potential for misinterpretation; an inability to cover the exhaustive moral content of medicine; and the lack of cultural sensitivity (Davis, 1996; Jeffery and Millard, 1997). Also, there are fears that this ideal approach is not fully appreciated in practice, and that doctors in particular, even if well-meaning in their paternalism, may over-step their defined remit, coercing patients into burdensome treatments.

Medical input to dying patients has many differing aspects. Though death may be a common end-point, the process of dying takes widely variable courses. These can require differing levels and types of input, from a variety of sources. A sudden unexpected death (e.g. a fatal myocardial infarction in a previously fit person) will have no 'medical' need for the patient, but the needs of the bereaved may be incredibly high. By contrast, a patient with a slowly progressive but highly symptomatic cancer could make heavy medical demands throughout their illness. Even within high levels of medical input, opposing philosophies in care of the dying are seen. Despite overlaps, the overall more aggressive approach of intensive care unit staff contrasts with the more conservative approach seen in palliative medicine. Both appear justifiable in their own setting, while remaining too different to come under a single label or a single judgement. The distinction stems from the essential 'likely benefit versus burden' analysis, which may justify the extreme measures employed to save the life of an otherwise healthy road traffic accident victim, but which may not be considered helpful to a frail patient with end-stage cancer. However, the clinical situation is never absolute and rarely so polarised (which will be expanded on later). The lack of neat distinctions means that a reliable embracing of a single medical approach is not possible. Though the apparent inconsistencies make criticism easy, it in no way reduces the importance of a medical role when applied appropriately, tailored to the individual needs and wishes of patients.

The remit of palliative care

In discussing the medicalisation of death it is important to review hospice and palliative care provision, which is increasingly shaping health care for the dying. Palliative care developed partly in response to the negative impact of over-medicalisation upon patients dying within depersonalised and technological health care settings (White, 1999). By allowing an acceptance that there can be a time when there is an inevitability of death, palliative care provides an alternative stance to those medical services and societies that regard death as something to be resisted, postponed or avoided at any cost (Clark, 2002). And by combining technical and humanistic approaches, patients can find greater dignity at the end of life; the right balance is an automatic product of patient-centred care (easy to find, but only if you look). Palliative care opens a middle path between chasing cure and acceptance of death – or perhaps offering a realistic combination of both approaches, 'to hope for the best and plan for the worst' concurrently. Crucially, by focusing primarily on the patient and not the underlying pathology, technical aspects of care are reduced to the minimum and tailored, so they are only pursued when they appear of sufficient benefit as perceived by the individual patient. Thus, palliative care sets out to reduce the 'over-medicalisation' and consequently should reduce most of the concern.

The hospice movement was formed to combat the acknowledged but unmet needs of many patients dying from cancer, particularly in the hospital setting, dating back to the 1950s. By listening to these patients and their families it was possible to highlight the diverse and complex problems that faced them (Saunders, 1998). Thus, contrary to preconceptions that a lack of life-prolonging treatments left no identifiable health care role, it appeared that a difference could be made to patients even close to death. And by the 1960s robust leading articles in leading medical journals were already highlighting terminal care (Clark, 2002). It also became clear that these patients' health care needs expanded beyond medicine to cover many disciplines including non-physical interventions, e.g. nursing, physical therapies, social work, psychology, and spiritual guidance. Consequently the hospice movement employed a multidisciplinary approach rather than the 'traditional' medical model, to address dying patients' needs and make the delivery of health care effective. It aimed to provide (Saunders, 1998):

- Learning and science of the mind
- Never-ending development
- Vulnerable friendship of the heart

Though medical input was included, it remained patient-centred and patient-led (emphasising dying patients' inherent worth and dignity) above the role of any of the contributing professional groups. This required a significant refocusing on the holistic approach, better appreciating the important interplay between physical, emotional, spiritual and social factors. In particular, the interdependency of mental and physical distress found within suffering leading to Cicely Saunders' concept of 'total pain' (Clark, 2002). It is acknowledged that without such a philosophical and ethical basis to care of the dying unacceptable patterns of practice could develop (Latimer, 1991). The potential problems include inadequate or unskilled communication of information; withdrawal of medical staff; patient labelling; and poor health care.

Subsequently these hospice principles, highlighting the merit of physical and psycho-social well-being, have been accepted as applicable to terminally ill patients and their families across all health care settings, with the more inclusive term 'palliative care' proposed in 1974 (Clark, 2002). Indeed, as an antidote to a blinkered biomedical focus, the palliative care 'approach' has provided a useful reminder of core health care values, applicable across all settings and all patient groups, not only required by dying patients.

'Dying' has been used here, for convenience but not correctness, to denote a patient in the later stages of an incurable illness as implied by 'the medicalisation of death'. However this subjective use of 'dying' is generally unhelpful and 'dying' is intentionally absent from definitions of palliative care ('terminal' is absent too, for similar reasons). We are all undeniably and inevitably edging closer to death, at different rates and with different levels of awareness. Conversely, all patients, whatever their condition, are still living until they die, and ideally living to the fullest. And so, without a clear distinction, patients should rarely warrant the label 'dying', except perhaps during their final hours or days, when 'dying' takes specific and necessary relevance.

Palliative care is now defined as an approach that improves the quality of life of patients and their families facing the problems associated with life-threatening illness (WHO, 2002). Specialist palliative care services have evolved from the hospice foundations to now cover a broader remit in ever-greater detail. Three tiers of palliative care have been described (see Table 4.1) that remain a useful outline to make the distinction between specialist and non-specialist provision (NHS Executive, 1996).

Table 4.1 Three tiers of palliative care to distinguish specialist from non-specialist palliative care provision (NHS Executive, 1996).

---

1. The palliative care approach
- Promoting both physical and psycho-social well-being throughout all clinical practice, focusing on:
  - Quality of life
  - Encompassing significant others
  - Respecting patient autonomy
  - Open sensitive communication

2. Palliative interventions
- Non-curative treatments aimed at relieving symptoms or improving quality of life by specialists outside of specialist palliative care:
  - Palliative radiotherapy/chemotherapy
  - Surgical procedures
  - Analgesic anaesthetic procedures

3. Specialist palliative care
- The active total care of patients with progressive far-advanced disease and limited prognosis and their families by a multi-professional team with recognised specialist training covering a broad mix of skills:
  - Medical and nursing care
  - Social work
  - Pastoral/spiritual care
  - Physiotherapy/occupational therapy
  - Pharmacy
  - Related specialities, e.g. psychology, and anaesthetics

Palliative care services focus on patients with life-threatening illness, when far-advanced progressive disease appears beyond curative treatment. In this palliative phase of an illness, quality of life becomes the overriding focus of care, either because no realistic disease-modifying treatments exist or because patients have chosen to opt out of available active treatment options. Palliative care aims to provide:

1. Individually tailored treatments to improve quality of life
   - Reduce symptoms, so patients feel as well as they can
   - Improve functioning, so patients do as much as they can
2. Information, support and guidance to patients around end-of-life decision-making
   - Enable patients to best direct their treatment plans
   - Enable patients to best direct their life/discussions

Though clearly prognoses in this palliative phase are generally limited, how limited is not defined, and prognosis can never be predicted for an individual patient with any meaningful confidence. Crucially, even if death is imminent, there is not a presumed need for all the patients in this palliative phase to require specialist medical input. All involved health care professionals, especially the primary health care team, hold an ongoing palliative care responsibility. In many cases this will fulfil all the palliative care needs of a terminally ill patient, without needing to be any more intrusive. In addition, specialists from other areas, such as oncology, complement this palliative care by providing specific palliative interventions such as palliative radiotherapy or chemotherapy, potentially alleviating the need for specialist palliative care services. Conversely, specialist palliative care can be just as pertinent early in the course of an illness (even if only briefly), as it is the need, rather than the timing, that is the key determinant of input. At present only about half of cancer patients appear to need specialist palliative input, which would predominantly be nursing advice and support.

Patients only require specialist input when specific 'additional' needs can be identified that appear manageable but beyond the scope of the patient themselves, their informal support and their usual health care professionals. Specifically specialist palliative care targets patients with 'life-threatening illnesses' or their families when experiencing quality of life or end-of-life issues that are sufficiently complex, unusual, or refractory to 'standard' managements that they require the attention of a specifically trained multi-professional team. Specialist palliative care provides comprehensive individualised assessments that allow targeted multi-modal treatments, comprehensive support and coordination of care. To be effective, specialist palliative care requires a broad-based health care team and sufficient time to address the complex and dynamic pathology; the polypharmacy; the barriers to assessment/communication; the multiple losses; and the marked uncertainty in an area with relatively little robust research on which to rely, numerous potential ethical pitfalls and often little or no time for second chances.

The presence of health care needs during a terminal illness is well recognised independently of medicine. National studies in the UK have revealed a need for increased palliative care services and resources (Addington-Hall and McCarthy, 1995). Impartial bodies such as NHS working parties have increasingly acknowledged the need for, and supported the expansion of, palliative care services to provide health care for dying patients across the UK, despite the high cost implications (Calman and Hine, 1995; NHS Executive, 1996; NICE, 2004). Moreover, even the staunchest of critics of the medicalisation of death can admit that palliative care has produced 'substantial achievements and significant benefits' (Field, 1994). These acknowledgements appear to justify, at least in part, a role for medicine in the care of the dying. This is also reflected in the rapid expansion of specialist palliative care worldwide (Higginson, 1998). It is harder to answer if the expansion palliative care matches only the already existing need or instead, by fuelling expectations and deskilling others, it could generate an increasing need for palliative care services.

Thus, assuming best medical and palliative care practice, Illich's original concerns could appear largely outdated, as historic anxieties may have been sufficiently addressed. Other factors now mediate some if not most of the original concerns (see Table 4.2). In particular, any subsequent technological advances have been countered by the increasing development and integration of the caring aspects of medicine. This facilitates a genuine choice for patients: an aggressive or a conservative management plan. Also, with explicit active treatment outcome tables and increasing rationing, rightly or wrongly acute services may now have reducing medical willingness to pursue relatively ineffective (arguably futile) treatment.

The potential benefits from a medical role in the care of dying patients

Health care plays an increasingly valuable role in the care of the dying. There are numerous and pervading benefits that can be identified:

- Proven benefits of specialist palliative care
- Accurate information that provides explanations and aids treatment choices
- Active treatment of underlying or concurrent disease(s)
- Relief from distressing symptoms

Table 4.2 Contemporary reflection on historical concerns around the medi-calisation of death.

Illich's historical critique	Contemporary view of shift since the 1970s
■ The loss of capacity to accept death and suffering as meaningful	■ Striving to survive is not a modern symptom, but central to evolution. There are now increasingly better treatments, with less toxicity and improved quality of life. Choosing to prolong life through proportional means is now easily justified
	■ Past acceptance of death may have reflected a desensitisation within a society faced with frequent exposure to death, with no alternative and thus not higher social values
■ A state of total war against death	■ Palliative care though part of 'medicalisation' supports reducing medical input to the minimum required or desired
	■ An increasing acceptance of death carries risks: the premature labelling of dying, the under-valuing of life, and potentially increasing society's tolerance for death from other causes e.g. road deaths or war casualties
■ The crippling of personal/family care devaluing rituals around dying	■ Though pain has a positive protective function (acute pain is valuable to warn and condition the body), any value is lost with chronic pain in end-stage disease, when any physiological or psychological benefit is absent... pain then becomes only negative
	■ Not all cancer patients will get pain... these patients are rightly considered fortunate, not disadvantaged by having a lesser symptom burden
	■ Pain and suffering can never be eradicated; despite all medical interventions patients will never get the chance to 'miss' out on pain and suffering
■ Society inappropriately viewing any rejection of the patient-role by the dying and bereaved as a deviance	■ Death is an unavoidable reality of nature, irrespective of all health care input. Patients fully realise this; closed awareness as a coping mechanism is not to be confused with a dysfunctional denial or lack of awareness
	■ Palliative care regards dying as a normal process (WHO, 2002) and supports the traditional family role wherever it can with increasing acceptance of palliative care input into 'mainstream' health care (NICE, 2004)
	■ Changes in society; dissolution of the extended family, globalisation and threats to the nuclear family (with more, particularly elderly, people living alone) have been supported by increasing mobility and modernisation. Thus the current modification of family values and rituals appear independent of medical advances. Health care has to be tailored to the here and now; and the shift is not likely to reverse, so rigidly looking to the past carries limited value

- Reassurance and inspiring confidence
- Respecting patient autonomy
- Respecting public opinion
- Empowerment of patients

- Provision of emotional support
- Mobilisation of related disciplines
- Lightening the 'burden' placed upon patients/relatives
- Bereavement support
- Potential for future improvements in care of the dying
- Additional indirect benefits of medical input

The proven benefits of specialist palliative care

There are numerous outcomes in care of the dying that that have been shown to be improved by adding a multi-professional specialist palliative care team onto conventional GP and hospital services (Higginson, 1998; Clark, 2002; Costantini *et al.*, 2003):

- Better control of pain and other symptoms
- More time spent at home, less time in hospital
- Improved patient and carer satisfaction
- Reduced overall costs
- Increased likelihood of dying in their preferred location
- Greater information on their condition
- Better communication skills
- Less likelihood of being admitted as an emergency, and less time in hospital

Similarly, as a result of increasingly robust evidence, NHS working parties have increasingly supported the development of palliative care services across the UK, despite the cost implications (Department of Health, 2004; NICE, 2004).

Accurate information that provides explanations and aids treatment choices

Following a detailed medical and/or nursing assessment, the cause of symptoms can be clarified (which may not be due to cancer or other established pathology, as is often wrongly assumed), and the patient's likely prognosis can be estimated. This will entail taking an illness history, an examination, and possibly investigations of the possible underlying pathologies. This medical information can prove invaluable in clarifying available treatment options appropriately and in providing explanations to patients, their carers, and other providers of health care. Without this insight, patients are disadvantaged, being less able to plan ahead or to make informed treatment choices or to enter meaningful discussions with loved ones.

Active treatment of underlying or concurrent disease(s)

Most would agree that medical input could be appropriate at one or more points of a terminal illness, e.g.:

- At diagnosis of a life-threatening disease
- At recurrence or disease progression
- At times of significant change in condition
- At times of physical and/or emotional suffering
- When death appears imminent
- The point of death
- Into bereavement

However, an acceptance of medical interventions restricted to such specific events is not practical. Key times can be described, but a terminal illness is a dynamic process, without convenient distinctions. If assumptions are made, mistakes and missed opportunities will follow. It can be argued that not offering available and proven therapies would be unethical and medically negligent. Thus, as medical input can be expected at some point(s) of a terminal illness, ongoing follow-up is advisable, even if only to exclude the need for any medical input at that time. This ensures continuity of care and maximises the possible benefits.

Even during a patient's final weeks the potential benefit of active treatment should not be underestimated. Oncological (for cancer patients), medical and surgical interventions can prove vital in treating the underlying pathology, any associated problems and concurrent disorders. A shift in focus in the role of chemotherapy over the last 20 years means that palliative chemotherapy can be shown to provide sufficient relief from tumour-related symptoms to offset the risk of treatment toxicities (Archer *et al.*, 1999). This will remain true for some patients with a presumed prognosis of only weeks or months. Such treatments may prove not only life-prolonging at this stage, but more importantly may improve the patient's overall quality of life. Even a few weeks of quality time may provide a priceless window to address previously 'unfinished business'. 'Active' treatments can range from simple antibiotic therapy for infections to aggressive or more interventional options. For cancer patients, these active options to palliate and/or prolong life include endocrine therapy; radiotherapy; cytotoxic chemotherapy; intra-luminal therapy (e.g. cryotherapy of endobronchial obstructions); and relatively major surgery, all of which can be surprisingly well tolerated and beneficial even in advanced disease (Thatcher *et al.*, 1995; Hardy, 1996; Gaze *et al.*, 1997; Maiwand, 1998; Middleton *et al.*, 1998; Rowell and Gleeson, 2002; Sze *et al.*, 2003; Patchell *et al.*, 2005; Wu *et al.*, 2006). A similarly broad range of treatment options remains available to patients deteriorating from non-cancer diagnoses. Patient choice appears pivotal. Patients would be denied these options if medical input were neglected. Indeed, patient groups are very vocal when limited resources restrict availability of desired active treatments (e.g. Herceptin seen as generating 'postcode lotteries' with geographical variations in provision).

It must also be remembered that dying patients are not spared concurrent illnesses, and have an enduring right of access to complete health care. Any coincidental medical problems will require appropriate attention. Good medical care must not be denied terminally ill patients as their condition deteriorates, based on unsubstantiated presumptions as to the cause and irreversibility of any decline.

Relief from distressing symptoms

There is abundant evidence that a large percentage of patients dying with advanced cancer or non-malignant diseases endure a high level of unpleasant symptoms (Vainio and Auvinen, 1996; Conill *et al.*, 1997; Addington-Hall, 1998). These areas of care need to be addressed. Health care forms the basis of symptom control – the appropriate medical/nursing input can alleviate pain and other distressing symptoms in dying patients. This can improve the quality of life, freeing patients to deal with more the productive issues of living, and to face their future even if limited. Pain, though perhaps the most feared symptom in cancer, can be readily controlled in most patients. The main reason for uncontrolled pain in cancer is inadequate management and not its refractory nature, as often thought. Similarly, realising the marked improvements in patients' quality of life delivered by some interventional treatments, such as intravenous rehydration and bisphosphonate infusions for hypercalcaemia, it is difficult to question medical advances, providing overall objectives of care are maintained (White, 1999). Effective symptom control needs to be a continuous process to ensure that care meets the current needs, reflecting the predictably progressive nature of terminal illnesses and their accompanying symptoms as well as likely changes in responses to medications. For instance, up-to-date reviews of any medications will allow drugs that are unlikely to be still conveying benefit or seemingly incurring side effects to be stopped, and other potentially more beneficial therapies offered if needed.

Reassurance and inspiring confidence

The communications revolution means we no longer live without at least partial knowledge, which can be dangerous and arguably prevents the 'ignorance is bliss' of patients in the past (if that was ever true?). Equally, changes in society mean that we are typically more self-determining and are expected to be responsible for our own health and well-being. These positive changes are double-edged; with increased responsibility comes a burden of accountability to oneself and others, which was previously ignored or abdicated to health care professionals. In failing health such vulnerability will be most evident.

Medical and nursing staff, trained in the care of the dying, can provide an invaluable source of support. The wealth of experience and knowledge gained can reassure and inspire confidence within patients, carers and other health care professionals. It provides an objective, evidence-based opinion to bring peace of mind to those who may otherwise feel like they are disadvantaged through being ill placed to deal with the relatively unknown. The existing structure of UK health care services means that every patient has 24 hour, seven days a week cover to provide equanimity. This is supported by specialist palliative care which has additional knowledge and skills in caring for the dying, and an increasing infrastructure to deliver it to all those in need. Some patients appear to require a medical presence, even without treatments, if only for the reassurance it can provide. At the other end of the spectrum, some patients may be disconcerted by any health care intrusion, even if arguably needed. There is no conflict: patients unconvinced of their need for medical input can simply opt out, as health care is always voluntary, available in case wanted. Of note is that there can be ambivalence in seemingly discontented patients: even patients who express concern at medical interventions to keep them alive when life has no meaning may simultaneously be worrying about dying (Holstein, 1997).

Respecting patient autonomy

Patient autonomy is the cornerstone of palliative care, realising its increased importance in end-stage disease. The doctor's role in providing information to help patients choose or refuse available treatments arguably enhances autonomy. Patients will be better informed of their disease and treatment options, including avenues of support to better direct their care and plan their life. Thus medical input should further empower patients to take charge and weigh the costs and benefits to define the individual level of medicalisation appropriate for themselves (Moynihan and Smith, 2002).

Thereafter, health care is obliged to respond and meet the high level of requests for care and support from patients with advanced diseases. Patients often appear dissatisfied when the active treatment options have run out. Such patients may demand further treatment, even surgery or cytotoxic chemotherapy, no matter how experimental, dubious, costly or far-flung. Treatments may follow on the basis of the patient's wish, possibly against medical advice, in search of a small, but real, chance of success.

Not only do dying patients court medical attention, but also (contrary to popular belief) they are happy to accept numerous invasive procedures and treatments (more readily than their nurses) (Meystre *et al.*, 1997) and agree to toxic treatments for relatively little gain (Griffiths and Beaver, 1997). Patients with cancer have been shown to be far more likely to opt for chemotherapy with a minimal chance of benefit than their professional carers (or people without cancer) (Slevin *et al.*, 1990). A more recent study in advanced cancer patients showed a wide variation in their willingness to accept chemotherapy, but with several patients happy to choose cytotoxic treatment for a survival benefit of as little as one week (Silvestri *et al.*, 1998). It is sometimes patients who are pushing for the right to have potentially futile treatments irrespective of best medical advice at the time (Re (Burke) v GMC, 2004), while at other times it may be the relatives (of patients lacking capacity) who would elect for more aggressive management rather than members of staff (Moe and Schroll, 1998). A demand for health care input even to dying patients is demonstrated by the large specialist palliative care caseloads, patients having requested or agreed to the medical/nursing input. A study of recently bereaved relatives revealed that 17% wished for greater access to physicians' time and nearly 10% had wished that further attempts at life-sustaining treatment had been pursued (Hanson *et al.*, 1997). In addition, it appears that, as death approaches, patients desire *more* formal rather than less formal medical care. In a study of their final two months, the percentage of cancer patients with their preferred place of care as home declined from over 90% to about 50%, the remainder wishing for hospice or even hospital care (Hinton, 1994a). Although this drop may reflect patients' fears of being a burden and the lack of available community support as much as any specific medical need, it remains persuasive that professional input for dying patients is currently both necessary and desired.

Respecting public opinion

The belief in a medical role in the care of the dying also appears to be reflected in public opinion, when considering the generous charitable support of independent hospices. If aggregated together, hospices would form the largest charity in the UK, receiving more than £100–150 million/year (Saunders, 1998; Tebbit, 2006). And the national provision of palliative care is increasing (Eve and Higginson, 2000). With such a clear endorsement, is the public wrong to seek specialist-supported health care once they develop a terminal illness? There is a need to respect such commonly held beliefs, which by definition conveys an ethical justification to provide palliative care services.

Empowerment of patients

A key component of any medical assessment is to determine a patient's expectations and aspirations from health care interventions. With this information, an existing knowledge of the available options and a communication network to access these options, medical staff are in a valuable position to act as the patient's advocate. By providing information and support, and acting on a patient's behalf, it should be possible to facilitate a patient's choices, for instance their wish to die at home (Seale *et al.*, 1997; Higginson, 1998), or their decision to discontinue cytotoxic therapy. Thus an increasing but appropriate medicalisation of death can paradoxically reduce the medical treatments a patient 'has' to face. Similarly the involvement of patients in their medical management may itself induce a sense of self-worth and determination, rather than it feeling like an imposition. Providing patients with a medicine to relieve their pain then allows them to become the victor, rather than the victim, over a symptom that may otherwise have served as a constant reminder of their illness and restricted their activities of daily living.

Provision of emotional support

Medicine and nursing can provide invaluable psychological support to patients, and more specifically develop coping mechanisms to help them face their diagnosis, which brings uncertainties, symptoms and losses. This can allow patients to find a level of comfort and spiritual ease that may not otherwise have been found. Thus the potential impact from external support during terminal illnesses and bereavement should not be underestimated. Though family and friends carry the key emotional support role, at times their vulnerability may limit their capacity to help. Frequently the presence of a trusted and familiar health care professional will enable patients to ventilate their feelings more fully, possibly for the first time, and without the fear of burdening family or friends. Also, an impartial opinion, particularly if suitably trained, can be a vital aid to reconciling potentially damaging family discord. More specifically, there is a high prevalence of depression in advanced cancer, which requires medical treatment as it can be highly responsive (in >80% of cases); yet depression is easily missed, even by doctors (Twycross, 1997).

Mobilisation of related disciplines

There is a role for medicine to support the 'non-medical' care of the dying. Though the palpable medical role may be limited, a significant role remains in facilitating care for patients from different professional or non-professional groups. A medical opinion may be influential in mobilising other relevant services, e.g. nursing, social services, therapies staff, complementary therapists, or input from a patient's spiritual guide. Such multi-professional input can be the key to maximising the care for dying patients.

Lightening the 'burden' placed upon relatives

The health care resource structure boasts an impressive array of assets that can prove invaluable to terminal patients. Medical, nursing, social services and therapies staff can access equipment and allocate packages of care to a patient's home, or facilitate suitable inpatient care. This practical support can lighten the 'burden' of care from relatives (and correspondingly lessen patients' guilt) or provide sanctuary for patients not wishing to die at home (e.g. to reduce distress for unprepared young children at home). More cancer patients and their carers wish to die in a hospice than might be expected (Thomas *et al.*, 2004).

Bereavement support

Medical input can be instrumental in identifying the need, accessing the necessary support, or helping directly in the management of difficult bereavements where concerns remain surrounding medical care; e.g. was everything done that could be? Why was the decline so rapid at the end?

Potential for future improvements in care of the dying

The formalisation of research and development within an academic framework such as medicine has led to better care for the dying. Medicine is constantly evolving, in particular the speciality of palliative medicine, which was only founded in 1987. Advances in palliative care have offered many patients a better quality of life through the control of pain and other symptoms, alongside attending to the different domains of their functioning. However, there is a lack of awareness of these new skills, and existing expectations of established treatments are erroneously low (both active and palliative treatment) with an inappropriately high acceptance of symptoms. Thus existing prejudices must be viewed with caution, particularly as they are often outdated and ill informed. It is essential that advances be disseminated through formal and informal education structures to ultimately make a difference to the majority of patients. However, there is still some way to go before all dying patients receive high-quality care, and improvements must continue (Addington-Hall and McCarthy, 1995; Addington-Hall, 1998).

Additional indirect benefits of medical input

Other unexpected benefits have followed the increasing role of health care in the care of the dying, for instance:

- The donation of organs such as corneas, tracheae and heart valves (Feuer, 1998). This can deliver a great sense of worth to dying patients and their relatives that surprises many, as well as the obvious benefits for the recipient of the organ. Sadly some have cited organ donation as a reason for concern, signalling the future 'inappropriate use of technology' (Field, 1994).
- The high profile of palliative care has led to the propagation of its core principles to other areas of health care, to reinforce the basics of good patient care.

Concluding thoughts

There has been a paralleling renaissance of the psycho-social aspects of care, which apply equally across all health care domains: quality of life; encompassing significant others; respecting patient autonomy; and open, sensitive communication. While medical values are improving (returning), sadly practice is lagging behind, and even being held back by limited resources. In the UK, over-stretched health care staff are increasingly forced to cut corners and focus on the most cost-effective and tangible aspects of care because of an increasingly results driven culture. Thus services with inadequate funding, as well as still having to meet NHS targets, will inevitably only be able to achieve the 'required' quantitative biomedical measures, at the expense of the 'desired' qualitative psycho-social aspects of care. This is a political and societal failing, which opposes current wisdom on good medical practice; it is unfair to lay the blame on health care professionals, who with adequate managerial and financial support would deliver the more rounded care they want to offer.

References

See the list of references at the end of Chapter 5.

An overview of the medicalisation of death, and the part played by palliative medicine

Part 2: Analysis of the potential drawbacks to medical input for dying patients

Craig Gannon

Introduction

It is feared that health care's increasingly comprehensive involvement with dying patients could generate, or even impose, expectations on society to die according to medical or nursing models. Once established, such expectations of medical input at and around death would be self-propagating. This increasing 'medical' dependence could limit individuals' expression, and divert attention from the real issues of death and dying. There is circumstantial evidence to support this argument, with acknowledged changes within society in its approach to death. Members of modern industrialised societies find death and dying hard to accept (Field, 1994). Though medicine has been implicated as having a causative role, this appears unlikely, as 'traditional' medical and nursing models are in fact constantly evolving in order to keep up with society's rising expectations of health care (General Medical Council, 1998). The resulting question 'Has society led medicine, or does medicine lead society?' can appear academic and impossible to resolve, with too many influences potentially accounting for the observed changes within society. However, critical reflection of the quantity and the nature of health care's involvement with dying patients remains essential to inform practice and service development.

There remain many different areas of concern that serve to question the appropriateness of health care interventions during terminal illnesses. Though they are addressed individually, for ease of discussion they overlap significantly, particularly the ethical aspects that touch all parts of health care practice:

- The increasing institutionalisation of death
- Unnecessary meddling in a natural process
- The undermining of patient autonomy
- Generalisations of care
- The detrimental effects of good practice
- Increased exposure to drugs and investigations
- The displacement of more relevant support
- The potential for poor medical and nursing care
- An unchecked (or unstoppable) drift from intended health care aims
- The potential impact on survival
- The additional burden of how and when to stop treatments
- Abuse of a privileged position
- Injustices in delivery of care

The increasing institutionalisation of death

An example of medicine's potential negative influence upon the dying is the increasing institutionalisation of death occurring within Western society (Hunt, 1997). Institutionalisation of death not only opposes patients' wishes, but the resulting care for patients dying in hospital appears lacking; described as dehumanised and socially isolated (Clark, 2002). Though 50% to 70% of patients wish to die in their own home, over the second half of the last century the percentage of home deaths has dropped in the UK from around 50% to only 26.6% (Higginson *et al.*, 1998). Patients in their final year of life occupy a quarter of hospital bed days in the UK (Clark, 2002). Consequently the average GP in the UK will now only care for two or three home cancer deaths a year. While historically the family doctor had an established and valued role in caring for the dying at home, many GPs can now lack the confidence to offer or encourage home deaths (compounded by inadequate resources and higher expectations of specialist services).

Similar statistics can be seen in other industrialised countries, such as France, where home deaths dropped from 64% in 1964 to 30% in 1983 (Rogue *et al.*, 1994), and South Australia where the proportion of home deaths has decreased continuously from 92% in 1875 to only 21% by 1990 (Hunt, 1997). These changes have fuelled fears that the increasing institutionalisation of death, within medicine and elsewhere, may be an irreversible process (McCue, 1995), and if the trend continues, home deaths could become as rare as home births (Field, 1994). However, it should be remembered that these figures don't reveal that 90% of all care during a patient's final year occurs at home (Doyle, 1998), and that the described decline in home deaths in England has actually halted since 1992, with a possible 'slight increase' in home deaths since then (Higginson *et al.*, 1998).

Importantly, quantitative data revealing low home death rates for cancer patients cannot be assumed to correlate directly to poor quality of care or the undermining of patient autonomy. To clarify any impact from, and the appropriateness of, hospice or hospital admission it is important to remember that patients' theoretical preferences on place of death may not match the actual choices they make on place of care when their death is potentially imminent. Thus, a better insight into the size and nature of the reported shortfall (of not meeting patients' preferred place of death) requires more subtle study:

- Each individual patient preference must be matched against their actual outcome
- Checking desired place of care immediately before death is most important, rather than desired place of death
- Review of the numerous competing positive and negative factors that influence patient choice of place of care immediately before death is required

The degree of realism informing patients' preferences for place of death can vary, from 'in an ideal world' mindset to overly pessimistic thinking. As this potentially undermines the weight of any preference, the underpinning reasoning needs to be explored; for example, patients may want the benefits of a home death or want to avoid the downsides of hospital care, or both simultaneously (Thomas *et al.*, 2004). Thus the framing, scope and timing of any question around preference of place of death can dramatically shift the results obtained. So, despite the political convenience offered by simply comparing public opinion or overall patient preferences with overall actual place of death statistics, such number crunching provides little benefit, locally or nationally, appearing 'data rich, but information poor'.

An uncomplicated decline in health that allows a patient to be maintained easily in the home environment, leading to a comfortable home death, is undoubtedly a common wish for patients and carers. However, this may not be the reality for everyone. Firstly, wishes may have to change when facing the reality of dying with complex needs at home. Secondly, a specific event requiring medical interventions may dictate the necessity for admission. Prospective follow-up of patients receiving ongoing hospice community team input showed that patients' preferences for inpatient care usually increased before or around admission (Hinton, 1994b). An investigation to test whether adequate home care could maintain comfort and help the adjustment of patients with terminal cancer did show the service was praised, but the 'realistic preference' for home care fell steadily from 100% to 54% for patients and 45% for relatives. Despite a far lower home death rate than originally hoped, changing preferences meant, when followed up, that most relatives approved of where these patients had received care and their place of death (Hinton, 1994a). While numerous factors may be argued as relevant, realising palliative care intervention was constant, and professional presence alone would not have appeared pivotal in reducing the wish to stay at home. Indeed, palliative care input has been shown to reduce the time patients spend in hospital, increasing their time at home (Higginson, 1998; Costantini *et al.*, 2003).

Qualitative research into preferred place of death in cancer patients and their carers has revealed a greater than expected wish to die in a hospice (Thomas *et al.*, 2004). The authors accepted that appreciation of this complex topic was still 'underdeveloped'. Thirteen factors shaping the place of death preference were identified, grouped into the informal care resource; management of the body; experience of services; and existential perspectives (see Table 5.1). This led the authors to review their stance on UK policy that currently favours home deaths, questioning the 'home is best' mantra.

Crucially, the reduction in home cancer deaths may represent a push from patients rather than any pull from medicine, redirecting the responsibility back to society and away from health care professionals. Modern families may not

Table 5.1 Factors shaping the place of death preference (Thomas *et al.*, 2004).

- Patient's social network and living arrangements
- Patient's assessment of the carer's capacity to care
- Patient concern for the welfare of the carer/family
- Carer's attitudes and willingness to care
- Symptom management
- Patient's fears of loss of dignity
- Patient and carer perceptions of the reliability of services and the degree of 'safety' they offer
- Patient's attitude to a hospice
- Patient's experience of hospitals
- Patient's knowledge and experience of community services
- Patient's attitude to nursing homes
- Patient's attitude to and outlook on, death and dying, including religious faith
- Previous personal experience of death and dying

be able to fulfil 'their responsibilities of care' (Field, 1994). This appears a consequence of changes in family and household structures such as smaller family size (with more people living alone), greater geographical spread, a higher proportion of working women, and the fragmentation of families through divorce, remarriage and cohabitation. This leaves deficiencies in the lay care available in the home setting. By contrast the need for lay carers has risen with the increasing life expectancy, which prolongs chronic illness, disability and handicap. This point is supported by the fact that in the UK older people and women were consistently less likely to die at home (Higginson *et al.*, 1998). Ironically, it may be under-, not over-medicalisation that has added to falling home deaths rates. On realising the increasing gaps in lay care, medical and social care have not expanded adequately to match the increasing need to allow patients to remain at home to die. Highly dependant patients may require 24-hour nursing care. Rationing of health care means that sufficiently high-level input is often not available in the patient's home. Similarly, limited resources may also reduce the availability or depth of cover available to patients at home from specialist palliative care services, with gaps in care (not patient need and not patient wishes) necessitating admission to a hospital or hospice.

Patients may fear dying at home either for themselves or their family. This can lead to patients actively seeking admission to a hospital or hospice as death approaches. These requests to not remain at home can arise from:

- The fear that their symptoms would not be adequately controlled at home
- The fear of being a physical burden on relatives as the need for care increases
- To spare loved ones the emotional pain and memory of a home death (particularly where young children are likely to be present)

Clearly medicine cannot be overly criticised for colluding in these aspects of 'the medicalisation of death', which may actually result from good care, respecting patients' wishes, or resource shortfalls outside of physicians' control.

Furthermore, for some patients, realising the scope of different needs and changing wishes, there can be justification for hospital being the most appropriate location to die. The patient may legitimately want continuing treatment and/or investigations even when time is potentially very short:

- Hospital-based expertise may be needed to deliver optimal symptom relief (e.g. radiotherapy or stenting for Superior Vena Cava Obstruction (SVCO) or ultrasound guided drainage of loculated pleural effusions or abdominal ascites). Even symptoms requiring less technical interventions, such as nausea and vomiting in bowel obstruction, can prove difficult in the domiciliary setting, necessitating admission.

- The nature and treatment of certain cancers (e.g. haematological and lymphatic malignancies) will make home deaths less likely (Higginson *et al.*, 1998). In this setting chemotherapy may be required even into the last month of life, and the potentially treatable acute complications of the disease, such as infection or haemorrhage, by prompting admission, may subsequently be the cause of a hospital death (Hunt, 1997).

- Even in advanced disease, patients may still want hospital admissions to exclude or treat potentially reversible pathology (e.g. a concurrent chest infection). Superimposed acute pathology cannot be dismissed as either good (the paternalistic concept of 'the old-man's friend') or untreatable; such generalisations cannot be defended. Bioethical principles still need to be followed with potentially life-sustaining treatments in patients' final months (Lam *et al.*, 2005). If a treatment offers a chance of net gain in health, that treatment must be offered, even if only as a trial, to clarify the risk–benefit profile (BMA, 2001). When an offer of active management that requires admission is taken up by a patient, it inescapably carries the risk of an institutionalised death if the patient fails to respond, declines rapidly, and becomes too ill to transfer back home.

Thus, it may be a genuine need or the unavoidable uncertainty around a terminally ill patient's prognosis that leads to unintended deaths occurring in hospital. Alternatively, the patient may not have reached a point in their illness that allows them to 'give up' on active management, such that they demand care in the acute hospital sector... just in case (possibly against medical opinion).

It is important to remember the practical advantages that hospitals provide and not merely dismiss a hospital death as inappropriate without consideration of the individual circumstances (Gannon, 1995). Hospitals can offer diagnostic services; 24 hour nursing and medical cover (to whom the patient may already be known); access to other specialist opinions; the flexibility of a large number of beds; and in many cases a location more accessible for visitors than the nearest hospice unit. These specific benefits should be considered alongside the expanding provision of hospital-based specialist palliative care (Hospice Information Service, 2006) that can increasingly deliver appropriate symptom control and support to dying patients in the hospital setting (Ellershaw *et al.*, 1995). A recent study confirmed that cancer patients admitted to hospital for symptom control had a significantly greater improvement in their symptoms if they received specialist palliative care (Jack *et al.*, 2003).

However, even hospital doctors acknowledge that for a considerable proportion (more than a quarter) of patients dying in hospital the location is not as appropriate as other places, such as home (Seamark *et al.*, 1995). Good medical care is obliged to be responsive to the individual needs of a dying person and should strive to correct this shortfall. Improvements are needed to allow a reduction of these hospital admissions, increasing the likelihood of a cancer patient's death occurring in a more appropriate setting (even if possibly still not at home) (Seamark *et al.*, 1995).

It can be argued that the increasingly appropriate shifts in medical input to dying patients is beginning to redress the imbalances of the past and significantly increase the proportion of home deaths again. Present health care initiatives to develop specialist palliative care and in particular home hospice services have been shown to deliver a relatively higher proportion of home deaths (Hunt, 1997; Higginson, 1998). 'Hospice at home' services expanded rapidly in the UK during the 1990s (Eve *et al.*, 1997). However, despite their promise, these services appear relatively expensive and convey limited impact. One study raised questions around cost effectiveness: it cost £5,121 per extra home death, with only 1 out of every 3 patients entering the service dying at home (Palmer *et al.*, 1998). Also, a recent randomised controlled study failed to show a benefit for terminally ill patients allocated to hospital at home, as they appeared no more likely to die at home than patients receiving standard care (Grande *et al.*, 1999). However, this failure may have related more to the generic difficulties within research in palliative care rather than a lack of benefit.

As unquestionable concern remains, there is a need for better services along the whole chain of events that could precede dying patients inappropriately receiving care in acute hospitals:

- Better community support to reduce crises
    - Improved primary health care team input
    - Improved specialist palliative care community team input, including hospice at home where affordable
    - Improved social care and equipment into the home
    - Better support for carers as well as patients – so better prepared mentally and physically for the reality of a home death
- Better responses to crises
    - Improved emergency/out-of-hours care; better continuity of medical care and easier access to necessary medications at home
    - Designated specialist palliative care community teams, free to respond rapidly
    - Rapid response of social care and equipment into the home
    - Better triage within hospital assessment units, with rapid but complete assessment in a suitable setting and timely transfers to more appropriate settings as needed
- Better alternatives to acute hospital admission
    - Rapid access to desirable nursing home placements
    - Community hospitals
    - Local hospice facilities, with capacity, i.e. beds and staff, resourced to respond rapidly

Moreover, it is dangerous to collectively label all admissions at the end of life as inappropriate institutionalisation. Such labelling could generate guilt or a sense of failure in those patients, carers or staff even when admission is genuinely needed in advanced disease, particularly when death follows as an inpatient. More worrying generalisations around the popular ideal of 'home deaths' could be used politically as a justification to under-resource needed inpatient palliative care within hospitals or hospices.

Unnecessary meddling in a natural process

Modern health care has been criticised as an unnecessary and artificial meddling in the natural process of dying. At first glance there appears reasonable justification for concern. As a society we now label dying as a time of suffering, resulting from an acute or serious chronic illness or injury. This 'preferred' concept reassuringly implies that death could yield to medical technology, thus denying the naturalness of death as an independent diagnosis consequent to old age (McCue, 1995). It is implied that such beliefs reflect the latest technological advances in medicine, having crossed natural boundaries to become detrimental. However, similar criticisms have been levelled at medicine for hundreds of years! Past medical advances (e.g. around sanitation, clean drinking water, antibiotics and immunisation) have impacted on dying to a far greater degree than most recent advances in medicine. And common sense tells us that present-day medicine will appear simplistic and even barbaric to future generations. We must not naively claim that medicine now has a control over nature that is anything more than steady progress along a continuum.

Moreover, even if Illich is right and modern medicine has edged past the point of no return, ending forever the concept of the natural death, on balance are we truly worse off? Was historical ignorance around the underlying mechanisms and current treatments of previously fatal conditions a better state for society, in providing fewer opportunities to intervene, and hence allowing more 'natural' deaths? Taking this to the extreme, in order to embrace the 'natural death', should we refuse to offer the latest medical expertise, even when knowing it will increase the number of:

- Babies dying during breech births?
- Pre-school children dying following road traffic accidents?
- Young adults dying from a straightforward chest infection?
- Women dying from breast cancer, possibly before both their parents?

In most settings, choosing to prolong life through proportional means, including medical interventions, could reflect nature's universal drive to live. Inherently, this fight for survival appears at least as well established and equally acceptable as any comfort with opting for an early death. Ultimately, death is an unavoidable reality of nature, irrespective of any/all medical input. While death itself is natural, satisfaction with dying sooner by choice may be argued as less 'natural', with the exception of patients faced only with burdensome treatments or patients in their final hours, days or weeks. Comfort with loss of life can occur for several reasons, when patients are:

- Tired with existence (either having lost direction and ambition, in need of better support, or possibly sufficiently contented, having completed all life's challenges satisfactorily)
- Tired of suffering (with symptoms, e.g. pain, depression or feeling isolated, that haven't been addressed adequately yet)
- Resigned that all treatment options have been fully explored/tried with clear insight into a rapid decline in health
- Expecting to pass on to a better place after death (though now of reducing relevance for many within increasingly secular societies)

Regardless, as the clock cannot be turned back, the priority is for society to better realise its current needs and then make the best use of the current health care options. Irrespective of any superficial approval or disapproval, we need to accept that roles have evolved for health care increasingly throughout our lives and then ensure only input of overall benefit is accepted/delivered. These roles for health care already extend from birth, through daily living (in disease prevention, e.g. healthy diets, occupational health, child development, sexual/ reproductive health and immunisation programmes), up till death and into bereavement. A wilful denial of these roles discards any potential benefit from medical input, and when voiced, could discourage others from seeking much needed help and support. For some time health care has had acknowledged expectations broader than many realised. In 1958, The World Health Organization (WHO) defined health as 'not only the absence of infirmity and disease but also a state of physical, mental and social well being' (WHO, 1958). Medicine has to remember to respect *care* as profoundly as *cure* (Holstein, 1997). With this we need to prevent the over-treatment and over-testing of 'modern medicine's' approach to the dying (McCue, 1995). This requires dissemination of the essential blend of science, caring and ethics, with the clarification of the limitations of available treatments. Though scepticism may remain as to the 'presumed and perceived' benefits of medicine's noticed expansion into everyday life (Field, 1994), the way forward has to be better outcome assessment to clarify the impact of medicine in these settings. And rather than debating a misleading expectation of regaining the lost 'natural' death, it should instead foster the ability for medicine to 'change gear' and become more accepting when death becomes inevitable. This will provide a basis for supporting any truly beneficial measures and refraining from any interventions that are futile, cannot be substantiated or are not desired.

Health care cannot be complacent, as any input inevitably converts people to patients. Patients may, under medical direction and supervision, become the worried unwell; not living to the fullest. Patients can become ruled by 'other people's fear' of their death, with disproportional and counterproductive worry to be robbed of self-control. Medicine can be battling against death without realising the importance of living life for the patient or all the negative consequences of medical intervention. Health care professionals may thus divert patients from self-care and self-determination (Hall, 2003). Though doctors want to inform patients, the use of indigestible medical statistics may serve only to confuse and mislead individual patients. Rather than getting on with whatever life brings, with the same uncertainties as the rest of the planet, once faced with stark median survival figures or bewildering relative risk values, patients may struggle to place such authoritarian information away in the back of their mind (while being unable to resist asking for statistics in the first place). Every symptom, even seemingly trivial aches or pains (seen as normal when fit and well) may create concern in health care professionals and consequently their patients. Defensive investigations can follow ('just in case') that will leave patients in an unhelpful state of constant alert. Patients asked to keep symptom diaries can be left transfixed by that day's score of, for example their pain, rather than focusing on more positive aspects of getting on with life. For those patients that live past their predicted survival based on median survival figures (which is by definition half of patients), every remaining day can feel like it will be their last; living on such borrowed time isn't living for most.

The undermining of patient autonomy

Although autonomy is a seemingly simple concept, the application of autonomy is not straightforward. The surprisingly imprecise nature of autonomy's role means that it is not absolute in clinical practice. Without black and white guidance, even genuine attempts to fully incorporate patient autonomy into decision making can unavoidably present health care professionals with uncertainty. For example, should the patient alone always decide: their best interests; the futility of treatments; the rationing of resources away from other patients; or the appropriateness of euthanasia; and then still decide, even when lacking capacity? As any decision is open to different opinions, an inevitable flexibility in applying autonomy can result. Unfortunately this flexibility also creates the potential for direct abuse of autonomy in both directions: overriding patients' choices or 'blindly' following patients' choices.

Despite the increasingly acknowledged importance of autonomy, it is still feared that doctors and nurses could take a paternalistic stance and undermine their patients' wishes (even if well motivated). This may involve undue professional influence on either treatment decisions or selective information exchanges. In particular, there is the fear that in advanced disease, medical input could lead to patients having to endure burdensome or futile treatment or enter into unwanted and distressing discussions about their disease. The 'medical control and manipulation' of cancer patients has been described as 'one of the most cruel forms of medicalization'. Patients may be pressured into quick decisions while still reeling from the impact of their diagnosis and overwhelmed by information and choices (Hall, 2003). Additionally, after accepting earlier medical input, patients can subsequently feel indebted to health care. Patients' gratitude and promises of further benefits inevitably generate a dependence on medicine. This may leave patients powerless to resist suggested health care interventions, even if unwanted.

While poor practice may leave bad experiences, medical input does not inevitably undermine patient autonomy. The increasing emphasis on respecting patient autonomy is a cornerstone of modern health care, particularly in palliative care. This has proved invaluable in addressing the undue paternalism of the previously medically dominant model of care. There has been a parallel power shift from the doctor to the patient. The doctor–patient relationship has become a more equal partnership, aided by the increasing value society places on self-determination and the communications revolution; typically the Internet can put up-to-date medical reviews at patients' fingertips as soon as they are available to their practitioners.

Palliative care further emphases the importance of patient autonomy (NHS Executive, 1996). As end-stage disease advances further, autonomy carries increasingly more weight compared to the other ethical domains. Patients' wishes remain 'absolute'; autonomy retains the same impact at all stages of the illness trajectory, including end-stage disease and even after capacity is lost. And recent changes to UK law now mean that patient autonomy is also supported after death around organ donation (HMSO, 2004). By comparison, the other ethical domains – beneficence, non-maleficence and justice – carry relatively less weight as death approaches. They lose influence as patients in end-stage disease move beyond aggressive/expensive treatment options; have a frailty requiring only better-tolerated options; have already poor and deteriorating health; and have a short prognosis. This reduces the size and duration of impact from attempts 'to do good' and reduces the potential size of any possible 'harm'. Similarly, as treatments are typically limited to comparatively cheaper options, investigations are used sparingly and there is no likelihood of longer-term recurring costs, there is a reduced risk of inappropriately diverting significant resources. All this leaves autonomy as the increasingly overriding ethical domain as death nears.

Reassuringly, any concerns that medicine would undermine patient autonomy seem mostly unfounded, as undermining patient autonomy would appear a clear abuse of power and not an inevitable consequence of medical input. All medical care for competent adults is initiated, agreed and continued by the patient. Thus the patient remains responsible for the nature and amount of any health care presence around their death, as at any other time.

- If all aspects of medical care are considered unpalatable, the patient merely has to avoid seeking medical advice.
- If only some components of medical care are not desired, the patient merely has to clarify which components are acceptable, and thereafter not comply with and not return to doctors unwilling to follow their specific wishes.
- Patients are entitled to seek as many second opinions as they see as necessary to get the health care they want. Indeed, despite not seeing eye-to-eye, this should be facilitated by the 'first opinion'. However, the availability of second opinions will normally be limited to local services and facilitated proportionally to the chance of success.
- A patient cannot be given any treatment without prior consent (excepting CPR in hospital, where consent is presumed until patients explicitly opt-out). Importantly, a patient can refuse any treatment or investigations and similarly refuse to enter into discussions, for any or no reason (rational or irrational), even if their refusal appears detrimental to their health. Medicine doesn't force discussion or coerce patients to comply with treatments (outside of the Mental Health Act, which then only covers mental health treatments) (Stationery Office, 1983). Equally, irrespective of any specific refusals, all other potentially beneficial treatments, investigations and information should still be available as required by a patient at any point in time.

The Declaration of Lisbon states, 'the patient has the right to accept or refuse treatment after receiving adequate information'. This right has been upheld by common law in the UK (Re B, 2002). Thus, even if a treatment conveys benefit, if it is administered without fully informed consent, health care workers risk a charge of battery or unlawful trespass. Equally, when patients lack capacity, their previously established wishes (as far as known and if applicable) have to be followed, as an unambiguous and informed advance refusal is as valid as a contemporaneous decision (Airedale NHS Trust v Bland, 1993; Re C, 1994). From 2007, this case law was cemented into statute in the UK when the Mental Capacity Act 2005 came into force, additionally allowing a patient to nominate a chosen proxy for medical decisions to further safeguard their health care choices if capacity is lost (HMSO, 2005).

Thus patient autonomy should not be lessened by health care interventions in advanced disease, except in cases of poor practice. Moreover, 'medicalisation' may increase patient autonomy by providing information and empowering patients' choices. By contrast, the legal protection in place in the UK is not yet seen worldwide. Until recently, in France the patient did not have the right to refuse 'artificial prolongation of life' (Rogue *et al.*, 1994). This privilege remained with the physician until 2005, when the law was changed to allow a conscious patient to refuse treatment for a life-threatening and terminal condition once fully aware of the consequences.

Patient autonomy can appear non-negotiable; autonomy has universally popular and legal endorsement. And at the end of life, autonomy is hallowed as the cornerstone of palliative care practice. However, in clinical practice many competing interests can dent autonomy's position. Defining the true extent of patient autonomy is not straightforward and autonomy cannot be viewed in isolation from the other ethical factors. Even legally, there are apparent inconsistencies in the weighting of autonomy, for example; patients can refuse but not demand treatment, while the legal imperative to follow patients' requests for treatments reduces specifically once capacity is lost (Samanta and Samanta, 2006).

Consequently, palliative care must question the pre-eminent status it places upon patient autonomy if it is to remain above criticism of contradictions in care (Farsides, 1998). Autonomy cannot be taken literally: it is subjective; it is dependant on external approval; and it has to be considered in the broader context. Autonomy must be distinguished from liberty, while its features of independence and sovereignty must not be over emphasised. Literally, autonomous decisions should only carry impact on one's self; but realising the connected-self (we do not live in total isolation) this is rarely possible. Furthermore, truly autonomous decisions appear impossible within health care decisions, as an impact on health care workers is unavoidable. Accordingly it can be appropriate for patients' choices to be guided by others, or sometimes for patients to even forgo independent choices, without necessarily compromising autonomy.

Definitions of autonomy typically emphasise the idea of a competent rational person making choices for reasons that reflect judgement and understanding (Farsides, 1998). Patients are judged as competent to make decisions provided they have specific capacity for that decision, at that time. However capacity is not 'all or none' as implied; it requires understanding, retention of information, a belief in all the information, balancing of both sides, and the ability to express a decision (HMSO, 2005; Watson *et al.*, 2005). For each of these subjective domains: what is the required level; which if any is more important; how can they be assessed; and who finally decides? We all sit on a spectrum of ability to give informed consent or refusal, having different knowledge, subjective values governing our lives and individual hopes influencing our choices. Terminal patients' fluctuating physical health, state of mind (including confusion and depression) and the potential influence of others, will further affect the quality of their decisions at any one time. So it appears impossible to discriminate objectively if a change to a dying patient's expressed wishes has sufficient capacity to need following to the letter or reflects a superficial and transient reaction better 'ignored', at least initially.

In addition, a balance has to be achieved between autonomy and other ethical values and principles (Farsides, 1998). Patients do not have an undeviating right to influence medical practice; rather, their views must be judged in conjunction with beneficence, non-maleficence and justice (as discussed earlier). As autonomy is not considered in isolation, there is scope for flexibility in ethically sound medical decision making. Arguably an unwavering adherence to autonomy is unlikely to benefit the patient, and may merely allow doctors to relinquish their medical responsibility. Are there stages in a terminal patient's decline when their autonomy moves from the power of choice, to becoming an unnecessary burden? Do patients really benefit from repeatedly being asked to face brutal truths, or to shoulder the responsibility for 'impossible' choices between clinically equivalent but statistically different treatments? Alternatively, does medical paternalism ever move from an abuse of power that strips patients of their rights, to being a considered humane action, sparing patients by carrying some responsibility from a better-informed perspective? Consequently, the required relative weighting of patient autonomy opposed to health care paternalism can vary over time and from patient to patient.

Inevitably, as patient autonomy is not always binding, a selective adherence to autonomy is possible. This flexibility can appear convenient for health care professionals; recruiting the patient's help to direct care when facing difficult decisions (shifting responsibility and blame to the patient), but not following patient's wishes when they don't sufficiently match health care expectations. Consequently, as the threshold at which patient autonomy applies is variable, doctors can use autonomy as the justification for letting patients jeopardise their health (by declining needed treatments or consenting to experimental drug trials or agreeing to an unsafe discharge), but at the same time autonomy can be ignored in patients genuinely trying to improve their health, e.g. wanting experimental drugs or CPR (if not seen as sufficiently cost-effective).

Ideally, only a duty to treat according to the patient's 'best interests' should sway health care professionals from respecting patient autonomy. But, in practice the underpinning motivation for health care professionals to follow or overrule autonomy is not simply the patient's clinical need for treatment (i.e. not the patient's 'best interests' alone). In reality a need to comply with the described legal precedents around treatment refusal and capacity, the availability of relevant resources, the needs of other patients and the level of both individual professional and organisational comfort with the patient's request (or refusal) will all impose upon autonomy. This approach appears to be both a legal necessity and common sense, but in part it also appears to be defensive practice.

Thus dogma based around autonomy being an absolute right cannot be defended, but this should not deter all possible measures to maximise the patient's contribution to end-of-life decision-making and thus reassure society against any concerns of over- or under-medicalisation. There are several clinical scenarios that require particular attention realising that patient autonomy may be undermined. It is crucial to clarify whether these represent an appropriate variance or unacceptable practice:

- Refusing patients' requests for treatment
- Rationing information provided to patients
- Refusing patients' wishes to stop treatment
- Caring for patients when lacking capacity

Even within best clinical and legal practice, double standards around patient autonomy are visible and potentially open to abuse:

- Patient consent must be sufficiently informed, but patient refusal can be comparatively uninformed.
  - Care can be diverted to 'compliant' patients – while the initially unclear, unsure or just scared patients who decline initial treatment can be left to fend for themselves, often discharged from follow-up, without sufficiently checking whether the patient's immediate refusal was truly or still what they wanted... sometimes only then to be reassessed when it is too late.
- If a patient agrees with their doctor, and the doctor follows that agreed plan, is this autonomy? Was the patient's wish pivotal or merely convenient?
  - Though autonomy may be implied as relevant, inconsistencies can be seen; for example a patient's refusal to reinsert an artificial feeding tube is more likely to be respected without question, than an equally valid request to remove such a tube. The omission feels more comfortable for staff spared the act of pulling out the tube, even though there is no ethical or moral distinction between an act and an omission (BMA, 2001), both carrying identical clinical outcomes.
- In practice a patient's refusal of treatment is effectively absolute, even if the refusal is likely to lead to serious harm. And a valid advance directive allows this autonomy to refuse treatments to continue unchanged should capacity be lost.
  - Even if they appear a patient's only way to avoid death, antibiotics cannot be given without consent, no matter how bizarre the reasoning or if the patient's understanding appears fairly limited.
- Though autonomy around treatment refusals is accepted as legally binding, it is still not actually absolute. This leads to ill-defined legal grey areas,

leaving health care practitioners at risk if the advice of the courts is not sought or not available.

- If a patient's refusal of treatment could put others at risk of harm (e.g. a patient with a contagious disease refusing isolation and treatment) that patient's autonomy can be overruled lawfully.

■ Autonomy is legally binding within treatment refusals but a patient's request for treatment is not always binding as effectively dependent on professional approval. Ironically, this means, in addition to criticism for over-treating patients, doctors are equally criticised for denying dying patients treatments. UK law has established that a patient cannot demand a treatment that is not seen as offering an affordable net gain according to their health care professionals and health care provider, ultimately remaining an issue of clinical discretion (R (Burke) v GMC, 2005; Rogers, R v Swindon NHS PCT, 2006). Although leaving the deciding health care professional comparatively vulnerable medico-legally, even requests for potentially beneficial treatment do not have to be granted if it is judged to deliver insufficient benefit, or appears potentially too dangerous (or 'intolerable') or too expensive (though rarely explicitly declared as the reason).

- Patients desiring one last chance at chemotherapy can be refused, even if some benefit is possible and even if the patient's request displayed sufficient understanding and reasoning. Yet, equally futile, equally dangerous and equally expensive drugs may be given to other patients, e.g. as part of a trial, with patient consent possibly founded in more limited understanding or bizarre reasoning.

■ Valid advance directives, though described as equivalent to contemporaneous competent requests, in fact only maintain autonomy for treatment refusals; the legal need to respect patients' already limited autonomy to request treatment is further compromised at the point when capacity is lost.

- Though a competent patient's request for artificial hydration and nutrition in advanced disease has to be followed, this is not so once capacity is lost, even with a valid advance directive requesting them (Samanta and Samanta, 2006).

Doctors remain obliged, ethically, morally, and legally to act in a patient's 'best interests' (Mason and McCall Smith, 1991). Yet once fully informed, patients would appear best placed to decide their own best interests. However, 'best interests' could appear to extend beyond autonomy. Thus potentially, doctors' selective adherence to autonomy could still be defended in terms of 'good practice' or 'the greater good', but it is difficult to separate the potential conflicts of interests involved, either professional or pecuniary. Refusing patients' requests when unquestionably misguided, e.g. a patient's wish to continue chemotherapy that has demonstrated no benefit only harm, appears a duty of care and not in breach of autonomy; the patient's wish is presumed to lack sufficient understanding. Good medical practice dictates that knowingly futile or burdensome treatments should not even be offered, let alone administered to patients. However, there are some within the medical profession who will be more willing than others to opt for treatments that appear less justifiable medically, following patient autonomy on 'compassionate' grounds. While this may appear 'kind', it could equally be seen as professionally weak (giving into pressure), and cannot be supported ethically when:

- There is no realistic hope of benefit (i.e. practice *without* an evidence base)
- Considering the likely harm, both physical (treatment side-effects) and emotional (lost time and collusion, which may prevent vital end-of-life discussions and social activities being pursued)
- Resources are wasted (Escalante *et al.*, 1997), both in health care time and drug costs, which are then denied other patients who could have benefited

However, 'best interests' still remains a subjective decision. In many cases, there will be differing opinions as to the presence or absence of potential benefit (particularly as psychosocial benefit can always be argued even when no physiological benefit is likely). And inevitably, discussions will be fuelled by the uncomfortable reality of finances. The willingness of doctors to meet patients' requests for expensive, toxic treatments with little chance of benefit appears higher in the UK private sector. Whether this more aggressive management is right or wrong is a matter of perspective; either the private sector is driven by 'fee attracting' activity or instead it is free from the unreasonable constraints imposed upon the public sector. Within any rationing, distributive justice is favoured ahead of both autonomy and 'best interests' in decision-making. As rationing disadvantages the individual, any dispute represents a health care provider–patient conflict and should never be seen as a doctor–patient conflict. While theoretically the courts, not doctors, should decide on ethical dilemmas such as the withholding and withdrawing of treatments, the practical limitations of the family courts in the UK mean that this can only be considered in a minority of cases where there is sufficient persisting disagreement (Samanta and Samanta, 2006).

The recent implementation of site-specific cancer multidisciplinary teams (MDT) within UK oncology services has brought in numerous benefits for patients (particularly equity of access to services and consistent comprehensive assessment); sadly the patient's role appears potentially compromised. Clinicians decide the provisional treatment plan in the MDT, without the patient being present in the discussions. Of these health care professionals, few if any will have ever seen the patient and most will not necessarily get to see the patient subsequently. It may be difficult for grateful patients offered such 'standardised' treatment plans to argue how it may not seem in their own perceived 'best interests'. A more autonomy-driven patient-focused model of MDT working has been described, where a cancer patient was given the opportunity to review all the different treatment modalities with each of the relevant treating physicians. Truly open, even critical, discussion followed, resulting in superior patient decision-making (Hall, 2003). This appeared a one-off (the patient was a member of staff), and while clearly desirable, the resource implications may prevent wider uptake in rationed services.

The potential need for balance between autonomy and paternalism is one of the most difficult dilemmas facing health care workers dealing with terminal patients, arguably more demanding than in other areas of care. Conflicts of interest can arise iñ hospices between patient autonomy and professionals' perceived duty of care, creating dilemmas around end-of-life treatment decisions. This is most evident when withdrawing life-sustaining treatment, e.g. stopping artificial ventilation, at a patient's request. Inevitably such an emotive request generates questions for professionals; what level and duration of consensus is needed before we can agree to stop ventilation, and then once agreed, when and how should we stop ventilation e.g. who turns off the ventilator and do we enforce a 'cooling off' period on patients beforehand? The factors that make such requests contentious stem from competing interests within health care decision-making that could detrimentally impact on patient care and patients' rights (Gannon, 2005a).

As already highlighted, medicalisation arguably improves patient autonomy. Indeed it is the impact of the disease that strips patients of their autonomy. By improving patients' symptoms and providing appropriate information and support, medicine can help patients to live closer to how they want to live. And specifically, by providing tailored information, medical input should further empower patients to take charge and weigh the costs and benefits of any medicalisation (Moynihan and Smith, 2002). However, as this medical information is subjective, any conflict of interest between physician and patient could corrupt this exchange. Patients may be swayed by doctor's professional or even personal opinions. The process of deciding the potential benefit of a medical treatment over the potential burden can be fraught for physicians as well as patients, as the expected scientific answer cannot be found, as the process lacks objective reference points. For example, a cancer patient's imminent death may not be obvious. As a result, aggressive anti-cancer treatment may mistakenly be offered and continued. Doctors cannot be held responsible for not having all the answers. Better models to aid the prediction of impending death, are needed to improve the data available on which to base end-of-life decisions (Escalante *et al.*, 1997).

Palliative care principles oppose collusion and strive for open communication. Indeed, most patients ask for full disclosure. Truth telling is crucial to all palliative care input and remains a valuable mantra. However, there may be occasions, for example delaying breaking of bad news in full, until a more opportune time, where the resulting sensitive deception or even temporary collusion could perceivably have a role within good practice. Discretion and appropriate timing could be seen as preferable to a non-thinking all-or-none approach. It is difficult to defend any blanket approach; absolute and instantaneous disclosure of all information or opting-out from giving any information.

Once started, it may be unhelpful to repeatedly push home the limited likely benefits of their palliative chemotherapy to a patient (as long as it is still being well tolerated) realising that there are clear benefits to the patient group as a whole. Does describing a cytotoxic treatment as having 'a 20% response rate' amount to deceit; is it a deliberately misleading account of 'an 80% chance of no benefit, just side-effects'? Or is this just inspiring confidence and fostering reasonable hope?

If someone wasn't even aware they had cancer, is it possible there could be an occasion when it would be apt to delay rushing in to divulge in full the bleak outlook of a disseminated malignancy? Is it wrong to wait until the right time (e.g. when all information including treatment options is available), or the right place (e.g. a quiet room, rather than the hospital entrance), or the right people are present (e.g. a patient's partner)?

It has been proposed that incorporating a 'practical patient autonomy model' will both protect the conscientious doctor and be in the patient's best overall interests (Garwin, 1998). The suggestions include:

- Early in the course of the doctor–patient relationship, the doctor should determine and document the patient's wishes regarding limits to future medical treatment.
- The doctor should initiate discussion of the full ramifications of a proposed treatment. This must include any potentially negative impact on end-of-life care, e.g. prolonged survival only in a comatose state or on life support systems. Studies suggest that patients are reassured and not terrified by these discussions, but will *expect* their doctor to open the topic.
- Encourage the patient to formally nominate and fully inform a legal surrogate (the necessary legislation became available across the UK in 2007, with the Mental Capacity Act 2005). There would then be an unquestionable point of reference should the patient lose capacity, from someone who was 'happy' to take the responsibility, prepared for the eventuality and properly informed. This appears a more effective course than written advance directives.
- If the patient imposes limits on treatment that the doctor finds ethically unacceptable, the doctor should decline to act as the patient's physician.
- Similarly if the patient finds the entire treatment plan proposed by one doctor unacceptable they should seek input elsewhere.

As described, autonomy's place is less clear once dying patients lose the ability to express their wishes. Advance directives help inform health care professionals, but even when appearing valid, they may not still apply fully. Advance directives also lack flexibility; patients lacking capacity are inevitably disadvantaged, as they lose the chance to change their mind as their situation changes. So staff may feel obliged to act as proxy for non-competent patients. Though this may be seen as a professional responsibility, there is concern that the patient's views may not be adequately represented. Care could reflect a single professional's own views or the institutional philosophy rather than any consensus of good care. And some relatives may not feel sufficiently empowered to voice any resistance to 'medical' decisions, let alone pursue their opposition sufficiently for it to be acted on. Before 2007, in the UK the next of kin had no legal jurisdiction over a non-competent patient's medical management. But since April 2007, UK patients have been able to appoint a 'designated decision-maker' with the legal backing to direct health and welfare decisions on their behalf in case they subsequently lose capacity (HMSO, 2005). Yet, patients may still not nominate their next-of-kin into this ('lasting powers of attorney' role), to spare their next-of-kin such a daunting role. It is expected that in most cases these nominated proxies will enhance advance directives (by fuller advance discussions) and provide a legal hierarchy (that is easier to defend legally). But a 'decision-maker' will not resolve conflicts between family members, friends and/or health care professionals. Ironically, it is only such areas of conflict that create any of the current dilemmas. As the new law has not yet been tested, it is not clear what should be done should conflict arise, e.g. if doctors agree with the next-of-kin, but both parties vehemently disagree with the nominated proxy's opinion of the patient's best interests. Thus, though the final responsibility for health care decisions is still meant to rest with the nominated lead clinician (even if the new legal picture implies otherwise) the changes may allow some doctors to opt out of this role 'unnoticed' (for fear of legal reprisals) and patient care may not always be better.

To 'safeguard' the patient's care, doctors and nurses remain legally obliged to act in a patient's best interests, whether they have capacity or not. In view of health care professionals' unique position, which combines knowledge, experience, objectivity, and patient intimacy, this remit appears a reasonable arrangement, with additional value once capacity is lost. However, it is not realistic or fair to suggest that this is flawless. Good practice for patients lacking capacity would demand an agreement of all involved parties: the patient's GP/district nurses; hospital staff; palliative care staff; and their family/significant others. And then any decision must be in accord with the patient's previously expressed wishes. Clearly such a broad consensus may not always be possible. Difficulties can arise from unmovable differences of opinion or more likely the practical limitations of maintaining the multiple contacts to reach agreement.

The validity of health care workers as a patient's proxy can be further questioned, as it is not uncommon for disagreements occur within a clinical team. The final responsibility for deciding best clinical management rests with the nominated lead clinician, who is typically a doctor. Although this is contentious for other health care professional groups, the medical remit is merely consensus-finding rather than actually deciding. Arguably the lead clinician is as well placed as anyone to carry this responsibility and has the necessary experience and training. Delegation of the role to another member of the team offers few advantages, with similar, if not more, limitations:

- Senior nurses (offering a different but no more valid opinion)
- More junior members of staff (who, though less experienced might know the patient better)
- An independent clinician (unbiased but comparatively unfamiliar with the case)
- The team's chief executive (lacking the clinical knowledge and carrying a financial agenda)
- The law courts (time-consuming, public, concerned with precedents as much as an individual's needs and emotionally and financially draining. The courts can only say what is excluded as unlawful... not what should be done within the lawful options)

Medical advocacy or family proxies will always be open to criticism, as any judgement of 'best interests' is open to question. A doctor's previous knowledge of the patient will never be absolute. Indeed, the continued erosion of the 'cradle to grave' approach within medicine may leave doctors increasingly disadvantaged to act as the patient's advocate. The vogue for increasingly large multidisciplinary and multi-professional teams can now leave patients without a clear lead clinician (Gannon, 2005b). Surprisingly, evidence suggests that family members are not necessarily a better proxy. Their knowledge of the patient's wishes may be equally limited, or obscured by personal opinion or grievances. Relatives can have misconceptions as to the patient's suffering (typically overestimating symptoms) or may be a poor proxy for reasons of covert or overt personal gain, e.g. financial or social.

The role of autonomy in euthanasia requests poses particular disquiet for many health care professionals. Palliative care's development in part served to counter support for euthanasia (Clark, 2002). But palliative care's collective resistance to the legalisation of voluntary active euthanasia appears to be at odds with reputed public opinion and potentially patient autonomy, as opposition it is not merely based on the legal constraints in the UK (NCHSPCS and APM, 1997a; George *et al.*, 2005). Undeniably, a number of requests will come from competent, informed people who would never be swayed from their belief that euthanasia was right for them. Conversely, it is common for hospice patients to have life-sustaining treatments stopped or not started at their request, i.e. passive euthanasia, a term that confuses more than it explains. At first glance, realising the lack of distinction between acts and omissions in ethical or moral terms (BMA, 2001), concurring with patients' requests for passive but not active euthanasia could appear as though palliative care will listen to patients' wishes only if they are in concordance with palliative care opinion. However, the situation is not so straightforward. Though palliative care may need to be sympathetic to requests and facilitate discussion of euthanasia, there remain many cardinal reasons for opposing the legalisation of euthanasia and physician-assisted suicide (PAS), and again patient autonomy is only one of many factors that need to be considered (NCHSPCS and APM, 1997a; George *et al.*, 2005). Indeed, euthanasia and PAS, in requiring assistance, could be considered outside of autonomy. However, palliative care must be more open in acknowledging the complexity of the ethics around euthanasia and PAS to prevent misconceptions, to avoid apparent contradictions in practice, and to aid in the practical management of clinical dilemmas. No one can judge euthanasia and/or PAS as either right or wrong. Right or wrong is merely a matter of perspective and we are all entitled to have our opinions (individually or collectively). The public, media and political debate is fuelled by equally justifiable moral, ethical, religious and philosophical arguments. The key question is not can euthanasia ever be seen as compassionate (as many would, even if unwillingly with many reservations, have to agree 'yes it can'). Rather, the question is 'will legalising euthanasia or PAS do more good than harm?'. On balance, any legalisation of euthanasia or PAS in the UK will do more harm than good, as the current law suffices in most cases; the proposals are too subjective and inconsistent, thus appearing unworkable and unsafe, and risking hasty and inappropriate action. Just as with capital punishment, despite popular support, legalisation elsewhere in the world, and moral justifications, euthanasia legalisation should not be supported in the UK. Additionally, if health care professionals are to be involved in legislation, they have to answer, 'is killing patients, or helping patients kill themselves, ever a treatment?'. Again here the answer is 'no'. Palliative care, like all areas of health care, may be required to oppose euthanasia and PAS on biomedical grounds, as no net gain in health is obtained and no specialist knowledge, skills or equipment are required. But the confusion that follows misplaced guilt and ignorance can cloud the picture for some health care professionals (having witnessed sub-optimal symptom control, having been party to inappropriate actions previously, or if there are just unnecessary concerns around withholding/withdrawing treatment and the doctrine of double effect).

Palliative care's opposition to euthanasia and PAS does not reduce patient autonomy; there are already several legal options available for patients committed to shortening their life:

- Patients can commit suicide; this is fully legal, and the necessary means and know-how have never been so available. Even life insurance will still typically be paid (if more than 6 months old).
- Current UK law and professional medical practice means that patients can stop/refuse any treatment – as discussed, this is legally binding and reassuringly patients can use advance directives to keep the same right to stop/refuse treatment if they were to lose capacity.
- Patients can voluntarily refuse food and fluids (VRFF). Unlike euthanasia and PAS, VRFF provides a fully autonomous and already legal route for patients wishing to end their lives, which still applies after they have lost capacity, through valid advance directives (Gannon, 2004a). VRFF is more effective, quicker and cheaper than euthanasia or PAS.

However, VRFF shares the same moral and clinical discomfort for clinicians as euthanasia and PAS. VRFF is not a treatment and health care professionals cannot suggest VRFF as an option to their patients. Yet palliative care is in no position to oppose the legality or morality of VRFF, realising that the patient's right to refuse treatment has to be upheld. Equally, any resistance to VRFF by supporters of PAS and euthanasia appears misplaced. Why is there a need to legalise another mechanism for dying? Seemingly euthanasia and PAS are fine (suffocation) but VRFF is unacceptable (dehydration). If patients are ready to be killed because of unbearable suffering, why all the fuss/illogical distinction around the mechanism, particularly realising the additional benefits of VRFF to the patient? Distress is no more likely from VRFF than euthanasia or PAS. Reassuring evidence and experience from palliative care suggests that patients can die comfortably without the need for artificial nutrition or hydration.

Generalisations of care

It is argued that any health care-based approach to the terminally ill will draw dying people into 'a system', to be processed as patients rather than remain individuals. At best this can only be defended in part. Generalisations specific to the health care setting can be seen, with a clear contrast evident in approach between hospital and hospice care services despite overlapping patients. Potentially, hospital may be too aggressive or hospices too conservative. While palliative care aims to provide individualised care, patient selection cannot sufficiently explain the discrepancy, with presumably scope to improve in both settings. While the adoption of palliative care principles in the hospital setting may improve the care for many patients, on occasion hospital physicians may be too quick to adopt a more conservative approach, which provides a seemingly acceptable alternative. Though the motivation for withdrawing active treatment will typically be well meaning, the timing could be influenced by competing agendas: to improve treatment outcomes, to reduce costs, or to divert stress-inducing patients to other services.

Inevitably in providing any service some generalisations will occur. Within well-organised teams of experienced and like-minded health care profession-als, 'routine' areas of care will occur. This will remain true even as death approaches, no matter how hard it is resisted. Even within specialist palliative care, which emphasises the importance of individualised patient-centred care, there have been criticisms of a pervading 'odour of goodness' (Maddocks, 1998a). There will always have to be compromises, for example:

- The rationing of resources – in offering a service to a population, it will inevitably be tailored to the greater rather than the individual good. This is particularly evident on busy, under-staffed units such as hospital surgi-cal wards, where there appears little scope for the high levels of attention needed to provide individualised care to the dying. Even hospices usually operate referral criteria to target those with the 'highest' need, despite the benefits that could be offered to other patient groups. And within 'qualify-ing' patients, hospices are rarely able to offer individual patients longer term inpatient stays (a rapid turnover is needed to meet the overall demand) or admission outside of normal working hours (when staffing levels are lower to save costs), even if potentially beneficial.
- The maintenance of a workable service – most hospices would not admit patients that weren't already known to or assessed by the service (in an attempt to minimise inappropriate admissions) and normative precedents could hamper the spontaneity and flexibility of staff (McNamara *et al.*, 1994). Tensions arise between the differing ideals within the hospice movement; the constituent professional groups; the individual palliative care services; and individual members of staff. As a result these ideals need to be compromised to reach common ground.
- Altering a person's care due to their impact on others – a disruptive patient or one with an unsightly, malodorous or infective condition (e.g. MRSA positive) may be moved, regardless of their wishes, in order to benefit other patients.
- Education and research – a large percentage of clinical staff's time is devoted to teaching and research. Though this delivers benefits across the board, a patient with clinical needs at the time of a teaching session may not get seen as promptly.
- Standardised care – the Liverpool care pathway (LCP) has been introduced to transfer the hospice model of care into other settings (Ellershaw, 2002; Ellershaw and Ward, 2003). The LCP is increasingly seen as best practice

for patients dying in hospital and it is increasingly used in community settings and some hospices. The LCP's success, both clinical and political, however, brings some concerns. Undoubtedly the LCP can greatly improve on poor practice in hospital, but it is not a substitute for specialist palliative care; similarly, the LCP is possibly not as suitable for use within specialist palliative care services. However helpful overall, the LCP does risk reducing care to a standard checklist of items, with the audit process adding to a real or perceived pressure on staff to minimise variances – moving to 'one size fits all' for convenience, rather than individualised 'tailor-made' care which requires more time and better trained staff to deliver. Unless carefully monitored, the LCP's increasing acceptance as the gold standard risks focusing on paperwork ahead of the patient and stifling development (of best care and of staff).

There are more worrying concerns that the consequence of generalisations could extend beyond the tolerable restraints of working practices. Since the start of palliative care, a preset concept of a 'good death' has figured as a unifying goal featuring being pain free; openly acknowledging imminent death; dying in the home with family and friends; aware and without conflict or unresolved business; as a time of growth; and in a manner reflecting personal preferences (Clark, 2002). This ideal may not suit everyone and may not be realistic, leading to false expectations followed by guilt and disappointment at failure at such an emotive time. There is also a fear that patients' deaths may increasingly be expected to be 'appropriate' or 'convenient' and eased towards a particular institution's or health care professional's concept of a good death. For instance, increasing anxiolytic or antipsychotic medications for their sedative side-effects could generate a picture closer to the 'good death' for hospice staff, but might disadvantage patients still wishing to explore potentially unfinished business. It has been argued that 'Making someone die in a way that others approve, but he believes a horrifying contradiction of his life is a devastating, odious form of tyranny' (Farsides, 1998). Unfortunately some hospice patients' needs don't sit easily with the service provided, although hopefully their care is rarely compromised. There is evidence that hospice nurses manage less well emotionally with patients who don't fit their preconceptions of a 'good death' (McNamara et al., 1994, 1995). This is of some concern, as who other than the patient can define the 'good death'? Further research shows that patients and palliative care workers differ in their conceptualisations of a 'good' death (Payne et al., 1996). The patients' descriptions of a 'good death' highlighted dying in one's sleep, quietly, with dignity, pain free and suddenly. The members of staff, in comparison, highlighted symptom control, family involvement, peacefulness and a lack of distress. A similar study of Australian hospice nurses suggested they believed a death to be 'good' if there was an awareness, acceptance and preparation by all those concerned (McNamara et *al.*, 1995). Difficulties can occur when patients only agree in part to the offered health care. Even though the refused component(s) of care may make up only a small proportion of the total care, it may nevertheless be considered vital to the staff involved. For instance, hospice inpatients may refuse analgesia on religious grounds, or because of a stoic personality, despite clearly escalating pain and explicit advice. This is difficult to witness and may compromise other aspects of care (e.g. avoidance of physical care for fear of precipitating more pain). However, this doesn't justify witnessed backlashes such as 'if they won't have pain relief they shouldn't be in a hospice'. Any attempt to protect staff members' perceptions of the patient's best interests ('we know best'), although well intentioned, sacrifices the patient's autonomy. As discussed, the implications of patient autonomy are not boundless; however, we must not be too conservative or restrictive if we are to remain true to the original individualised philosophy of palliative care (Farsides, 1998). To ensure optimal development, there is a need for research programmes into death using different methods (including advance consent and qualitative approaches) that focus on the patient experience (Clark, 2003). Better training, adequate staff support and sufficient resources to allow flexibility in provision of care should minimise unnecessary generalisations. In contrast, we must also acknowledge that generalisations may not always be inappropriate. Though individualised care is promoted as central to palliative care, we should also admit that it coexists with the 'generalisations' of evidence-based practice and ethical and professional principles.

The detrimental effects of good practice

Even within best practice, inadvertent detrimental effects could arise from professional interventions. Tangible health problems such as drug toxicity (as below) or health care acquired infections will inevitably occur as a result of medical input. Equally, health care will generate harmful psychosocial consequences. A health care role around the time of death may fuel unrealistic expectations and lead to increased dependency within patients and society.

It would appear that both medical services and society are content to assume that every cause of death can be resisted, postponed or avoided (Clark, 2002). A mutually beneficial collusion of denial could fuel the medicalisation of dying, creating false hopes, such as expectations of cure. This collusion is a dangerous and destructive cycle that could impair the process of acceptance of the inevitability of death. These fears now seem largely outdated, relating to the collusion found within the medical practices of the 1950s and 1960s (Field, 1994). The withholding of information from a terminally ill patient is now rarely seen and long acknowledged as bad practice (Buckman, 1996; Seale *et al.*, 1997). However, even in palliative care, where open discussion is expected, euphemisms are still used to cover up painful realities and inflate possible outcomes to foster hope:

- The term 'good death' is used; but the 'least bad' death is more applicable.
- 'Impeccable assessment' is expected (WHO, 2002); but at times, rushed assessments from under-resourced services, with managers advising 'cutting corners' is inevitable, even within the best provision.
- 'Holistic' care is advertised for what has reduced to predominantly 'physical' care (Clark, 2002).
- 'Multi-professional' care is expected; yet 'mono-professional', predominantly nursing, care is delivered.
- 'Urgent symptom control' label for hospice admissions; when used for a rapid decline where 'urgent terminal care' looked more likely. A recent study confirmed that more than 70% of 'urgent symptom control' hospice admissions died during that admission, mostly within two weeks, and they outnumbered the number of hospice deaths admitted with the label 'terminal care' (Gannon, 2005c).
- Hospice admissions are optimistically arranged for 'symptom control' of even chronic refractory symptoms such as pain, when actually meaning last-ditch attempts with specific drug and non-drug interventions (that necessitate admission), hoping at best to 'partially reduce some symptoms in some patients'. Clearly if a quick fix really was possible on admission, it would have been tried earlier, probably at home.

Thus palliative care development may fuel impossible expectations on the effectiveness of symptom control in particular. Some symptoms, including pain, particularly incident bone/neuropathic pain unresponsive to round-the-clock and as-required opioids, will often prove refractory; moreover many symptoms will inevitably increase as patients deteriorate further (e.g. weakness, anorexia and breathlessness). In this setting, management focuses on providing supportive care to mitigate the impact of these symptoms rather than any 'control' as such. Moreover, many symptoms, such as sadness and suffering, cannot be 'fixed', appearing unsuitable for medical management (Macleod and Schumacher, 1999).

Unfortunately many patients admitted for 'symptom control', as well as their families, are disappointed on arrival at a hospice when simple effective options are not suddenly available and they can appear unprepared for what often becomes a terminal admission that feels anything but 'good'. Frequently community staff will have arranged such hospice admissions when simply 'stuck', without identifying the cause of symptoms (e.g. as potentially dying or superimposed reversible acute pathology) and are then left unable to identify any additional interventions that could possibly improve the refractory symptoms. This appears dishonest, being either overly optimistic or just using admission as a convenient option to compensate for unacknowledged limitations within the community services. Typically such an admission follows the need for the sanctuary of 24-hour generic nursing care when a patient is dying or at an equally difficult time for carers, where 'psychosocial crisis' is a more apt label than 'symptom control', even if it doesn't sufficiently fit expectations. While labelling is primarily the subject of academic debate, misinformation from casual terminology can prove detrimental to care; it is important to prevent inadvertent collusion by misuse of the category 'symptom control'. Patients, families and hospice staff may all be tempted to aspire for the impossible, particularly in advanced disease when the reality may feel too uncomfortable for many to accept in advance. Fuelling false hopes must be avoided: an equal struggle will follow the disappointment of treatment failures, even (and possibly more so) if subsequently the hopes were realised to be unrealistic.

For example, as a result of this misplaced shared optimism, hospice inpatient stays may be unduly prolonged (until patients become 'well enough for discharge'), further increasing disappointment when this proves unobtainable. Postponing such a discharge usually leaves the patient with advancing disease less well placed to be discharged: the delay increases dependence; allows the background disease to progress further; and increases the patient's exposure to the potential toxicities of drugs. Rapid opioid dose escalation is the commonest example of iatrogenic harm; higher opioid doses can still be pursued, despite the lack of a clear dose-response, seemingly out of desperation/blind hope. Each therapeutic failure increases the conviction in the next attempt, despite dwindling likelihood of benefit. Thus the delay forms a vicious circle, making a discharge home increasingly difficult. Consequently, patients may be discharged to residential or nursing homes rather than their own home or perhaps achieve a discharge home but at a point in their illness when they are less able to enjoy it.

Patients may develop a dependence on health care in general, in a specific team, or in an individual professional. This could act as a barrier to communication within a family, add emotional strain or resentment, or allow family members to distance themselves from care and from facing the realities of death. This could reinforce and perpetuate a death-denying approach. However, this need not be the case. As highlighted, palliative care values the role and needs of dying patients' family members. Appropriate palliative care, besides helping patients cope better, should facilitate their relatives' needs and care roles to ensure that both parties are better prepared to face the impending death more positively and more realistically. Conversely, medical input will expose patients to the harsh realities of median survival figures and their potential disease trajectory, in order to inform balanced treatment decisions. While generating 'false hopes' or denying patients requested medical details clearly appears misplaced, if some patients feel better able to cope when 'blissfully unaware' (not knowing either way), this state may offer more to their quality of life than having clarification of what may appear to be 'no hope' at all. For a number of patients (even if a small minority) that aren't yet able to take in bad news constructively, any medical disclosure, by increasing awareness without the necessary acceptance being possible, may be equally or more distressing than being unaware.

On a broader scale it is argued that there is a general and expanding dependence of modern industrial societies upon medical care to solve all their problems (Field, 1994). As a result it is claimed that there is a reduction in the ability to cope with pain and suffering (Illich, 1990). However, this diminished ability for people to manage or to cope with their own health appears to reflect industrialised societies' high expectations with an increasing need for support across various walks of life, increasing the dependence on identifiable organisations (the council, employers, the police, the government etc.). Instead of marginalising medicine, we should provide education to skill the general public in shouldering all life's responsibilities, such as their health and how to relate positively to authoritarian organisations.

Increased exposure to drugs and investigations

Over the last 20 years in particular, advances in palliative oncology (Archer *et al.*, 1999) and palliative care (Twycross *et al.*, 2002) means there are an increasing number of appropriate drug interventions that can be offered to patients with advanced or end-stage disease. Inevitably, the risk of futile treatment persists within both active medical management and palliative care. Of concern is that reports continue to back this worry: 47% of advanced cancer and dementia patients in an American hospital study received invasive non-palliative treatments in their final days and the SUPPORT study described a 'medical juggernaut... less focused on human suffering and dignity than on the struggle to maintain vital functions' (Clark, 2002).

The expanding palliative care presence in terminal care has led to a growth in possible pharmacological interventions with an increased risk of inducing side effects, allergic reactions and drug interactions. Particularly feared are the highly toxic effects of most chemotherapeutic agents, which could appear to counteract their therapeutic value in the palliative care setting. However, the picture is not that straightforward. A relatively recent study of women undergoing high dose chemotherapy for metastatic breast cancer (with severe side effects) did not demonstrate any measurable reduction in their quality of life as might have been expected from a toxic treatment. Instead, this chemotherapy regimen afforded patients the chance of increased survival and the prevention or delay of disease-related symptoms (Griffiths and Beaver, 1997).

Another fear is that sedation could follow the use of drugs such as painkillers, clouding the patient's consciousness and thus impairing their quality of life. Paradoxically the opposite appears true. Good analgesia with morphine can actually improve psychomotor functioning (e.g. driving skills). Reassuringly, the importance of potential adverse effects from drugs is realised in palliative care, and these are carefully monitored, discussed with patients and if deemed significant (or not manageable by other means) the offending drugs would be discontinued. This highly attentive approach should ironically reduce unwanted drug effects experienced by terminally ill patients, despite the utilisation of medications. Over recent years increasing medical attention has led to the more judicious use of drugs, such as forsaking the Brompton Cocktail (a mixture of morphine and cocaine, in alcohol, syrup and chloroform water) (Ashby, 1998) and avoiding the previously 'heavy-handed' approaches to increasing morphine dosages.

Similarly the importance of non-pharmacological interventions in symptom control is now far better realised and readily utilised to allow the minimisation of drug therapies. Complementary therapies (e.g. acupuncture, aromatherapy and art therapy) have an expanding role within palliative care. Specialist palliative care services and even UK cancer centres are increasingly providing access to complementary therapies as a core part of their remit (Clover and Kassab, 1998; Kite *et al.*, 1998).

Patients have additional safeguards against inappropriate exposure to drugs and investigations. All medical interventions must potentially provide a net benefit and then they can only be pursued with the individual patient's explicit agreement (as above). Doctors should not even offer, let alone start, knowingly burdensome or futile treatment, investigations or information exchanges.

The displacement of more relevant support

Any health care professional role in the care of dying patients risks diverting attention from more appropriate formal and informal channels of support. In particular, it is argued that increasing specialist palliative provision to patients at the end of life brings the unnecessary intrusion of strangers into the home and hampers any established health care provision. Though undeniable in part, in practice these concerns may not prove as bad as feared. Specialist palliative care input aims to complement and maximise the care available to patients. The advent of specialist involvement does not negate the need for, or necessarily undermine any other support systems available to dying patients. In fact, specialist palliative care should bolster patients' existing support mechanisms.

Just the presence of health care workers could be seen as harmful during the period leading to a person's death. The involvement of 'strangers' could appear intrusive during this private family time. Patients and their families may feel obliged to disclose personal information and allow access into their homes. Many patients or their families may be uncomfortable with personal care being delivered by health care professionals. This loss of control, privacy and dignity could appear as yet more losses above the numerous losses that typify a terminal illness. Thus, for a number of patients, lay carers and non-health care professionals will be better placed to comfort them when death draws close and the 'traditional' role of medicine is reduced.

Palliative care sets out to utilise all potential sources of support in order to benefit the patient, which may not include a need for any ongoing medical input. It is increasingly common for specialist palliative care teams to refer patients back just to their general practitioner's care when a specific need can no longer be identified. Regardless, the patient is encouraged to follow the most suitable line(s) of support (e.g. family, friends, spiritual leaders and/or self-help groups). There should never be any routine health care provision to dying patients. Medicine's regard for the role of non-professional carers in supporting terminally ill patients is seen in the ongoing research into the collective wisdom of lay people who were familiar with dying and death (Donnelly, 1999).

When professional health care support is required, continuity of carers with named key-workers can go some way to lessening the concerns for patients and their families. And though continuity is a priority in health care (particularly palliative care), this is not practical on a 24-hour, all year round basis. Even with the best continuity of staff, this is only an answer in part; involving a consistent member of staff outside of the patient's circle of family and friends at such an emotive time, will still present issues. If there is a clash of personalities (which may be missed if subtle) the patient or family may dread the health care professional's arrival. Alternatively, 'special' bonds between staff and patients could be seen as undermining family relationships, adding to the feelings of inadequacy common in relatives watching a loved one's relentless decline. Moreover, physical intimacy, such as handholding or sensitive touch, even when delivered in a balanced professional manner, could be construed as inappropriate.

There is also anxiety within fellow health care professionals, in that the increasing medical presence in the care of dying patients is unnecessary and hampers existing provision (Fordham *et al.*, 1998). The increasing involvement of specialist palliative care in terminal care has generated professional concerns surrounding continuity of care and professional responsibility and accountability issues, e.g.

- The role of lead clinician becomes confused
- Increased patient uncertainty with conflicting management plans
- Increased breakdowns in communication from increased numbers of involved personnel reducing continuity
- The increased risk of deskilling non-specialist health care professionals, who remain responsible for the majority of care, for the majority of patients
- Uncertainty around specialist palliative care's multidisciplinary working (in particular the advisory role of specialist nurses), with a belief that any expertise is exaggerated or unscientific (Maddocks, 1998b)

However, concerns that specialist palliative care inevitably hampers the established health care provision to dying patients appear misplaced, merely reflecting generic issues of the generalist–specialist and specialist–specialist interfaces, which will be especially prominent with any new specialty. Health care professionals outside of palliative care may not fully appreciate the specialist clinical care that can be provided. GPs and hospital consultants may be unfairly critical of palliative care if they are feeling threatened (Maddocks, 1998b) or merely unaware of the nature of or the value of the evolving specialist knowledge that overlaps into their domains. Generalists may also be less familiar with the non-clinical aspects of the specialist remit that justify the expansion of specialist palliative care. Education, research, advice and training future specialists would also be lost if specialism in care of the dying were suppressed, as would the resource generation that funds the vast majority of inpatient hospice care in the UK.

This limited insight within non-specialist health care workers may reduce their confidence in specialist palliative care. Some health care workers have limited awareness of even basic symptom control measures, failing to achieve as effective symptom relief in their terminal patients (with other outcomes appearing less favourable too) and with possibly little information on when to refer for help. This suggests a need for more specialist palliative care with better training in palliative care (Addington-Hall and McCarthy, 1995; Ellershaw *et al.*, 1995; Morrison and Morris, 1995; Barclay *et al.*, 1997; Grande *et al.*, 1997; Higginson, 1998). Thus specialist palliative care provides much needed extra experience, knowledge, skills and resources to support non-specialist provision. As with other specialties, few problems should or do occur in practice with good cooperation in individual cases and a greater overall acceptance should follow as palliative medicine continues to integrate into mainstream medicine (clinically and academically). It is worth reiterating that many studies have validated a role for adding specialist palliative care to conventional services for dying patients (Higginson, 1998). The merit of multiprofessional and multidisciplinary teamwork between specialists and generalists is generally accepted, appearing commonplace across all areas of health care, including the community setting (e.g. home assessments with follow-up from community psychiatric nurses with consultant psychiatrist support).

Consequently, specialist palliative care makes communication and education covering, patients, their carers, and other health care professionals a priority. Palliative care provision has already increased into hospital outpatients and inpatients, obtaining earlier referrals, liaising with primary health care teams, and taking up formal teaching opportunities at undergraduate and postgraduate levels. Teaching programmes should ensure the specialist wisdom gained is passed on so as to further skill, and not deskill, non-specialists.

Admittedly there is a lack of clarity around palliative medicine's remit, as distinct from terminal care, hospice care or palliative care (Field, 1994). Specialists have been accused of failing to adequately define what they do and how it differs from other health care areas (Clark, 2002). As a result of unclear terminology, inevitable overlaps, ongoing evolution and the unusual situation of a specialty that primarily relates to the impact of an illness, not the stage or underlying pathology, palliative care definitions can lack clarity. Subsequent misunderstandings could curb attempts at professional cooperation. Indeed, with marked variations in service provision even in the UK, the definitive aims of palliative care do not appear universally verified. However, as described, clear and workable definitions of palliative care are available, internationally (WHO, 2002) and nationally (NCHSPCS, 1995; NHS Executive, 1996), while specific local guidelines can usually be obtained from service providers. While some details within these definitions will still differ, this is inevitable as palliative care evolves, and this mark of adaptation should not be viewed as a failing. Indeed the lack of clarity of definitions reflects the 'beauty' of palliative care, in that it isn't restricted to a specific disease or life stage (Lapum, 2003). And palliative care provision will continue to be better defined as it matures. Currently, patients with 'life-threatening illnesses' require specialist palliative care input when they or their family present with unusual, complex or refractory quality of life or end-of-life issues, which cannot be adequately managed within non-specialist provision (i.e. when primary care and other specialties need help). Ultimately, there is a shared responsibility for specialist palliative care to inform other health care professionals (and the public) of their services, and equally for all professionals caring for terminally ill patients to find out what specialist palliative care could offer their patients.

The potential for poor medical and nursing care

Although good care is the intention of any health care provision, there is a risk that poor care may inadvertently be delivered to dying patients. The structure and processes within health care systems may negatively impinge on the quality of care for some patients: for example if care is rationed (reducing staff numbers or training); standardised (as above); or directed towards quantitative rather than qualitative targets. Consequently mistakes may be made, causing harm to patients (e.g. drug errors or misplaced alarm around MRSA). However, any occasional bad practice needs to be eliminated and not used as an excuse to condemn all medical practice and foil the good work that does take place.

Inevitably health care involvement risks suboptimal and on occasion even poor care being delivered to dying patients. The causes behind problems with care will be varied, but they will more commonly follow system errors rather than an individual health care professional's sole error. Increasing steps to improve the quality of health care systems and eliminate poor practice are in being put in place. In the UK in the late 1990s, the National Health Service (NHS) introduced 'clinical governance', a managerial framework, required by law, to ensure that financial control, service performance and clinical quality were fully integrated at every level within 'well-managed' health care organisations (Scally and Donaldson, 1998). Clinical governance brought a statutory duty for NHS organisations to formally seek quality. Each NHS organisation had to demonstrate the provision, coordination, monitoring and responses to the numerous and diverse professional and organisational quality initiatives required by their service (local and national). Clinical governance committees were formed to oversee or link into the National Institute for Clinical Excellence (NICE); The Health Care Commission; clinical effectiveness/audit/ quality assurance; risk management/health and safety; staff development (e.g. recruitment, selection, Continuing Medical Education and revalidation); user involvement/complaints procedures; and clinical research. Clinical governance's overview of the various systems clarified the responsibilities for quality in health care (who should be doing what, so fewer gaps and fewer overlaps) and clarified the accountability for quality in health care (who is to blame if care goes wrong).

But compromises in health care provision are unavoidable. The increasing costs of health care and increasing litigation have fuelled political drives in the UK to focus on easily measured targets around the quantity of health care (rather than the quality of health care); a defensive focus on reducing poor practice (to reduce litigation) without promoting excellence (as improving best practice is rarely as cost-effective in the short term); and standardising clinical input within increasingly large multidisciplinary and multi-professional teams (a tick-box rather than free-thinking culture) (Gannon, 2005b). Medical progress has created increasingly complex care for dying patients, needing the involvement of an increased number of different specialist medical teams, often spread across several sites. Limited resources mean that hands-on care is often delegated to more junior grades (correctly, in part, called 'training') and to other, less 'expensive' professional groups (correctly, in part, called 'team-work'). The resulting reduction in clear medical 'ownership' of a patient can undermine continuity of care and increase the chance of oversights (Gannon, 2005b). Though we can now show we are doing more, more quickly, and the National Health Service has sufficient clinical documentation for a robust defence in court, are UK patients actually getting better care?

Even within 'best practice' perceivably inferior care, even if still accomplished, will occur at the tail end of the spectrum. Studies have highlighted the need for better communication skills and better symptom relief in the care of the dying (Addington-Hall and McCarthy, 1995; Hanson *et al.*, 1997). Health care professional involvement around the time of death also brings the potential for more untoward interventions. This may result from the subjective nature of many of the complex clinical decisions within terminal illnesses (as differences of opinion will occur) or less comfortably from a lack of knowledge, experience or willingness to follow good practice. Bad practice may be fostered by misdirected attempts to help or direct abuse. This ranges from genuine mistakes, including inappropriate therapies offered with well-meaning intentions ('the doctor knows best'), to the coercion of patients for the personal gratification of health care workers (e.g. research projects based on financial or career development issues rather than clinical grounds). A study in America concluded that some physicians might inappropriately use their medical prerogative to protect their professional autonomy. It appeared that extreme legal defensiveness could significantly influence some physicians' assessments of medical futility, such that they would wish to pursue predictably futile treatments irrespective of the lack of any potential gain to the patient. In this situation a conflict between the physicians' interests and terminally ill patients' own end-of-life decisions can be anticipated (Swanson and McCrary, 1996).

Improvements in medical education and research will increase the awareness of care of the dying, and allow practice to continue improving. Audit needs to be in place to check that best practice is being followed. Additionally, despite the numerous difficulties, sound ethical research is a key component if any real progress is to be made, as research provides the evidence to improve upon current best practice (Gannon, 2004b). Although dying patients appear particularly vulnerable, research should not be feared on ethical grounds. Palliative care patients are just as deserving and possibly more in need of the attention and subsequent benefits of active medical research. With the expansion of pharmacological treatments within terminal care there is an acknowledged demand for rigorous evidence of effectiveness (Ahmedzai, 1997). Reassuringly, any research already requires rigorous and independent ethical approval, and patients must be fully informed and consenting. And importantly, many dying patients appreciate the chance to participate in research. Arguably health care professionals should practice evidence-seeking as well as evidence-based practice.

Important progress is being made, with the voluntary hospice movement being heralded as an example, from which 'the NHS can learn' (Department of Health, 1998). Other shifts in care have happened, to improve the medical/ nursing practice provided to terminal patients. In oncology a marked change in research methods, from a fixed focus on survival figures after treatment, to recognise the need for and incorporate quality of life measures, to allow more holistic assessments (Thatcher *et al.*, 1995; Hardy, 1996; Gaze *et al.*, 1997; Maiwand, 1998; Middleton *et al.*, 1998; Rowell and Gleeson, 2002; Sze *et al.*, 2003; Patchell *et al.*, 2005; Wu *et al.*, 2006). Similarly, there have been marked improvements in communication between doctors and their patients with cancer (Buckman, 1996). In repeated studies in the UK between 1969 and 1990 there has been a significant increase in open as opposed to closed aware-ness of impending death. As a result, the patients and relatives were more satisfied with their degree of choice over place of death, were less likely to die alone, and more likely to die in their own homes (Seale *et al.*, 1997).

An unchecked (or unstoppable) drift from intended health care aims

The increasing acceptability of medicine and nursing input in terminal care runs the risk that any evolving direction taken by health care may deviate from its intended or agreed objectives. It is feared that unacceptable health care interventions could insidiously become the norm. Thus the ongoing develop-ment of palliative care is entering a risky phase (Clark, 2002), with the poten-tial to drift from its original intentions in its care for the dying. Some argue that palliative care has already lost some of its original motivating spirit. Compro-mises have followed the encroachment of mainstream medicine into palliative care with its technological imperative to investigate and treat, its professional empowerment (particularly medical), disease-centred practice, evidence-based practice and the need to conform to rigid standards and limited budgets (John-son *et al.*, 1990; McNamara *et al.*, 1994; Bradshaw, 1996; Maddocks, 1998a; Hoy, 1999; White, 1999). The original hospice philosophy 'disapproved' of the care given in hospitals to dying patients (seen as burdensome and intervention-ist) and aimed to return patients to their own home to die. Yet palliative care is now responsible for a multiplying range of interventions for dying patients, and rather than increasing the percentage of home deaths, in the main there appears to have been a movement of deaths from the hospital setting to another institution, the hospice (Higginson *et al.*, 1998). Additionally, while palliative care's goal of improving quality of life is impressively holistic, in reality there is an increasing emphasis on physical symptoms ahead of any psychosocial concerns (Clark, 2002). Specialists in palliative care are feared to be evolving into 'symptomologists', drawn by the biomedical model and a focus on randomised controlled trials skewed towards physical symptoms – the palliative care team at an Australian teaching hospital, in listing 24 problems, described only two that were not physical (depression and delirium). Similarly, a multinational study of symptom prevalence highlighted the physical symptoms of pain, nausea and dyspnoea, and offered only one non-physical symptom, confusion, in its commonest nine symptoms (Vainio and Auvinen, 1996). And there has been a parallel shift towards greater medical intervention, such as invasive procedures, which has appeared with little questioning or exploration of the causes (White, 1999). This medical encroachment, in competing with the original 'good death' ideal, has also been linked to tensions within the multidisciplinary team (McNamara *et al.*, 1994).

It has been acknowledged that one of the challenges facing palliative care is to address the trend towards medicalisation (Corner and Dunlop, 1997). However, any shift in palliative care provision may not be as undesirable as is sometimes implied. It may represent:

- Advances in available medical and nursing care offering, on balance, sufficient improvements in dying patients' quality of life to justify the interventions
- Increasingly complex clinical needs, within longer-term survivors because of greater natural reserves and more effective active treatments
- Changes in society's structure, reducing the informal support networks: a growing number of single person households (as many as a quarter in many European countries), decreasing family size, broken bonds through divorce and increasing employment for women (Jordhoy and Grande, 2006)
- A response to the ever-increasing expectations of patients

As specialist palliative care broadens to include patients ever earlier in the course of their terminal illnesses, integrating with curative and rehabilitation therapies, there is the potential for a reciprocal decrease in focus on patients' last days or weeks and terminal care to become marginalised within palliative care (Field, 1994), with a diminished emphasis on the good death (Clark, 2002). These concerns are difficult to dispute, and talk of 'the greater good' and 'equity', may sound unconvincing to those within palliative care driven by ideals of 'final care'. However, the increased availability of palliative care should not necessarily impact adversely on terminal care provided adequate resources are made available. Indeed, the rapid expansion of palliative care seen in the UK has recently had a significant additional NHS contribution, so a marked dilution of existing services to complete the broadened remit has not been seen. This may not be continued; a 'fit' and 'sustainable' NHS may not be happy (or able) to fund specialist palliative care, possibly expecting charitable services to fill the void.

The potential impact on survival

There are fears that medical input may either hasten death or artificially prolong life. Reassuringly there is no evidence to support these claims for patients receiving palliative care. Indeed, the lack of any intention is highlighted within the WHO definition that states, 'palliative care intends neither to hasten or postpone death' (WHO, 2002). But an absolute lack of an effect on prognosis from palliative care input, in either direction, is impossible to prove. It would be unethical to run randomised trials in an attempt to find out whether palliative care did indeed influence survival (Ashby, 1998). In addition, palliative care patients may still require acute medical interventions. Treatments for hypercalcaemia, anaemia and infections are commonly provided in hospices and carry a potential to prolong life, even if this was not the overriding intention. And decisions around the withholding or withdrawing of such treatments, or in some cases, artificial nutrition and hydration, are clearly likely to impact on survival. Importantly, intentional steps to artificially shorten patients' lives are not part of palliative care. Ironically, some critics of the medicalisation of death see the artificial ending of a patient's life by an unnatural medical act, euthanasia, as a way of avoiding medicalisation! Sadly, but unnecessarily, this is seen by some as the only way to avoid burdensome life-prolonging treatment. In truth, as already discussed, patients can refuse any treatment, whether considered burdensome or not. By contrast many observers have confused palliative care with euthanasia (Maddocks, 1998b), despite palliative care having dissociated itself from the practice (Ashby, 1998).

There are specific ethical questions raised by health care's seemingly inconsistent approach to nutrition and hydration in the terminally ill. On one hand it is argued that dehydration can cause patient morbidity (e.g. thirst) and hasten death (Craig, 1994, 1996). In contrast, others believe artificial hydration or alimentation to be inappropriate in the terminal setting (Ashby and Stoffell, 1991). The available, albeit limited, data suggests that artificial nutrition and hydration have no influence on symptoms or survival when death is imminent (NCHSPCS and APM, 1997c). At this late stage, additional fluids are not related to, and thus cannot help, any reported thirst (perhaps as, often, an isotonic dehydration occurs) and similarly extra nutrition cannot deliver any benefits in terms of energy, weight gain or improved prognosis in patients faced with an extreme catabolic state. Moreover, any attempts at parenteral hydration (Dunphy, 1995) and nutrition in the terminal phase could have detrimental effects, for example fuelling false hopes; distressing pooling of fluid (in respiratory and gastrointestinal tracts); pain at site of entry; and the introduction of a physical 'barrier' distancing relatives.

The outcome of the differing views is that terminally ill patients in the acute care setting will usually receive intravenous rehydration, while those admitted to a hospice or remaining at home would not be artificially hydrated (Dunphy et al., 1995; Craig, 1996). Such discrepancies are hard to justify and do not inspire confidence in medicine's ability as a whole to act appropriately in the care of the dying. The reason for this quandary is the persistent lack of definitive research sufficient to overturn historical presumptions. Until this is found, it is likely that medicine will continue to divide into the two camps of 'standard' management. In the meantime we must admit our uncertainty, make individualised decisions, not prejudgements, remembering to elicit and treat any reversible causes of dehydration (e.g. hypercalcaemia), and be responsive to the wishes of the patient and their family (Dunlop et al., 1995; Dunphy et al., 1995). A recent consensus document summarises the current knowledge base to provide a framework for good practice (NCHSPCS and APM, 1997c). As always, the way forward is further research to provide sufficiently substantive data to unite medicine in its management of terminal dehydration. In the interim, the issues of artificial nutrition and hydration at the end of life remain within the constraints of withholding and withdrawing any medical intervention (as discussed below) and it is unnecessary and misleading to make a 'special' case for artificial nutrition and hydration.

A similar divergence of opinion and practice is seen in another emotive area, cardiopulmonary resuscitation (CPR) for the terminally ill. While the issue of CPR at the end of life principally remains within the constraints of withholding and withdrawing treatments, the default position of 'implied consent' separates CPR from all other medical interventions, so it is necessary to make a 'special' case for CPR, at least in part. In recent years great strides in understanding and practice around CPR decisions have been made in the UK. This has followed consensus statements (NCHSPCS and APM, 1997b; BMA, 2002), fuelled by national directives (Calman, 1992). However, CPR guidelines, as a necessary simplification, still contain significant concerns around patient autonomy, quality of life judgments and the role of families in decision making (Boyd, 2001). Indeed, there is still considerable variance in practice between hospitals and hospices.

In the hospital setting, irrespective of their condition, patients will remain for resuscitation from the point of their arrival until the issue of whether to resuscitate is discussed (if at all). As inevitably many hospital patients will have advanced disease, this 'opt out' policy within hospitals will lead to a higher number of futile attempts at resuscitation than desirable. By contrast, historically patients admitted to many hospices would not even be considered for resuscitation as standard practice; equally CPR would rarely be discussed or documented (Dunphy and Randall, 1997). And hospices do not normally have the skilled staff or equipment to offer advanced life support. Yet hospices are now admitting patients far earlier in the course of their illness, when resuscitation could be of value, and successful resuscitation in a hospice has been described (Noble et al., 2000). Thus the previously common blanket approach, to never offer even basic resuscitation, is now easily open to challenge. But even the use of an 'opt in' policy, unless supported by a robust pre-admission discussion and selection, means that some hospice patients may be denied desired resuscitation which, not unreasonably in a health care setting, they might have been expecting, even if highly unlikely to be beneficial.

Despite the overlaps, the 'opt out' policy for resuscitation seen in hospital and the 'opt in' policy for hospices would seem appropriate default positions for the majority of cases, realising the different patient groups and the different settings:

- Desire for resuscitation. Patients are in part self-selecting and in part professionally directed into hospice or hospital groups appropriately. Most patients admitted to a hospice would consequently wish for more conservative supportive care and actively want to avoid aggressive, arguably burdensome, acute hospital style care, such as CPR, and vice versa.
- Likely response to resuscitation. There is good evidence that CPR in the setting of advanced disease such as metastatic cancer or end-stage non-cancer diagnoses is unlikely to ever be successful, effectively covering nearly all hospice inpatients.
- Different clinical environment. On-site equipment and staff training in hospices cannot match the intensive care possible with the sophisticated facilities and specialist-trained staff in hospitals.

Consequently, successful resuscitation appears far more likely in hospital than in hospices; estimates suggest a more than 15-fold greater success in hospital (Thorns and Ellershaw, 1999). Thus, realising that this equates to less than 1% chance of success in hospices, few if any hospice patients would be disadvantaged by an 'opt in' policy. Regardless, as these issues are now well recognised and with implementation of the mentioned guidelines, practice should continue to improve in both hospital and hospice settings. Similar attention must also be given to terminally ill patients in the domiciliary setting where doctor-and-patient agreed anticipatory decisions on resuscitation, need to be recorded and communicated to any designated nursing or medical cover (e.g. G.P. deputising services), ambulance services and of course all carers.

The role of medications such as opioids, anxiolytics and/or antipsychotics, which carry sedative side effects, can also take on a specific ethical perspective when used for their sedative properties. A dangerous precedent can appear to be set whatever is done, with medicine over-stepping its boundaries if heavy sedation is prescribed, or acting barbarically if relief is denied to an imminently dying patient by withholding sedatives. However, these widespread fears of ethical dilemmas and even dubious practice appear overplayed. It is crucial to separate symptom control and transient sedation, which both appear relatively free from ethical controversy, and the more uncertain practice of 'total sedation', which can be difficult to distinguish from euthanasia. For example benzodiazepines can be used at different doses for different effects:

- Symptom control: for anxiety, muscle spasm, or epilepsy (where sedation is avoided)
- Symptom control: terminal restlessness (where sedation, though not desired, may be unavoidable)
- Transient sedation: as night sedation for insomnia; to cover specific procedures such as manual rectal evacuations of faeces; or for a crisis, e.g. a potentially terminal carotid bleed (where sedation is brief)
- Ongoing total sedation: purposefully rendering and keeping a patient unconscious with an expected shortening of life

It is normal in palliative care to use analgesic, anxiolytic and/or antipsychotic medications to relieve the symptoms of terminal restlessness during a patient's final hours or days, where sedation, though not desired, appears a common consequence. Any ethical concern in this setting appears misplaced, as the drugs are required for symptom control and no shortening of survival occurs. However, by contrast, sedating a patient who is not dying to the point of coma for an indefinite period to relieve refractory symptoms is of great ethical concern and is not part of normal palliative care (Ashby, 1998).

This may be an over-simplistic view of sedation at the end of life. These distinctions for sedation are not as clearly understood or described in practice and there are inevitable overlaps. An international, multi-centred study suggested that intentional sedation rates were as high as 15% to 36% at the end of life, most commonly for delirium, but most worryingly it included family distress as an indication (Fainsinger et al., 2000). However, the lack of a formal definition of sedation in the study plus the uncertain basis of the described 'intent' may fuel confusion and exaggerate the figures; was the sedation truly desired (purposefully using 'excessive' doses) or merely realised as a probable consequence of treating the symptoms (when using the lowest possible doses)?

When death approaches with distressing symptoms that appear refractory to all targeted measures, the role of sedation as a part of symptom control may have to be accepted. Indeed, offering opioids, anxiolytics and/or antipsychotics at the end of life when required to combat symptoms appears mandatory. Reassuringly this is not as difficult an area as often described. Following appropriate assessment, the conservative use of any drugs targeted against specific symptoms at the end of life can be considered ethical, even if unavoidable sedation follows as a side effect, as all the available data confirms that titrated symptom control measures will not shorten survival. Thus the fears of shortening patients' lives with symptom control drugs such as morphine appear misplaced, being based on outdated assumptions and beliefs from forty years ago (Maddocks, 1998b). This is particularly true of legal deliberations that, despite advice to the contrary, continue with the morphine causation myth (Ashby, 1998). Comfortingly, current best evidence confirms that neither opioids nor sedatives appear to hasten death when administered as part of appropriate palliative care (Sykes and Thorns, 2003a,b). Even if the quality or the generalisability of this evidence base is questioned, particularly in individual cases, the use of medications with sedative side effects would still appear ethical because of the Doctrine of Double Effect (DDE); legally the cause of death would remain the underlying condition.

Though not needed, the DDE provides additional 'protection' to cover any historical and theoretical concerns. The DDE states that a bad effect of treatment, even a patient's death, may be permissible if it is not intended and occurs as a side effect of a beneficial action (Thorns, 1998b). As described, the DDE should not need to be evoked for appropriate symptom control in terminal care, instead appearing more applicable to situations such as chemotherapy-induced neutropenic sepsis failing to respond to optimised antibiotic treatment. Moreover, it is important to stress that the DDE must be applied with care and accuracy. Misleadingly, it has been claimed that the DDE maintains 'a climate of fear and secrecy' with 'grey ethical principles' (Corner, 1997). However, the same author then employed it incorrectly, jumping from the relief of symptoms with the unintended risk of death, to intentional killing as a 'welcome secondary consequence' (Thorns, 1998a). This improper use of 'DDE' as a label to legitimise poor clinical judgements outside of its defined context cannot be condoned. The DDE has several safeguards to protect against abuse:

- The act must be morally good, i.e. in response to suffering.
- The doctor's intention must only be the good effect (the bad effect may be foreseen as a possibility, but never intended). Though intention may appear impossible to ascertain, a 'common sense' review of the drugs, doses and routes chosen are sufficient to judge intent (Forbes and Huxtable, 2006).
- The bad effect must not be the means of achieving the good effect (so a patient's death cannot be used as the means to relieve their distress).
- On balance the good effect must outweigh the bad effect (known as proportionality).

Though end-of-life decisions pose inherent difficulties, the DDE provides a helpful framework to reassure health care professionals, while concerns as to its abuse appear unfounded providing the above criteria are met (Thorns, 1998b). Additional legal advice in Canada has added, to similar guidelines, the need for documentation and a progression of any dose increases (Ashby, 1998).

Unfortunately, inconsistencies in the approach to sedation for refractory symptoms are visible. The Canadian Special Senate Committee on euthanasia and assisted suicide received a consensus from witnesses that the practice of 'total sedation' (i.e. rendering a patient totally unconscious) was widespread (Ashby,

1998). Similar cases have been openly discussed in palliative care journals where death could not otherwise be predicted as imminent (Shaiova, 1998). However, these appear to be exceptional cases and at odds with UK palliative care practice. The use of such heavy sedation is overrun with difficulties, such as confirming the refractory nature of the symptom(s) and the apparent end-stage of the patient's illness, as well as achieving a consensus of all involved parties (the patient, the family/carers, and other health care professionals). This practice remains highly controversial and questionable in view of the lack of any distinction from euthanasia in consequentialist or non-consequentialist terms (seemingly only separated academically by causation) (Ashby, 1998). Moreover, the DDE would not be applicable, despite arguably well-meaning 'hopes' that it could apply.

Of note for patients requiring ongoing symptom control medications that appear to be causing significant ongoing sedation, is that it is actually the lack of hydration, nutrition and ventilatory support that leads to any shortening of life, not the sedation itself. This provides further reassurance to prescribers that they can ensure their patients receive adequate symptom control without fear of reprisals. Thus, if it is feared that sedation may have shortened a patient's life, besides the evidence base confirming that sedatives do not shorten life in terminal care and the extra 'cover' provided by the DDE, the key ethical issue is still not 'Was the sedation right or wrong?' but 'Was the withholding of the vital supporting treatments right?'. Additionally, clinical rules have been described to better safeguard decision-making to prevent the indiscreet use of indefinite heavy sedation (Cherney, 1998):

- Symptoms should only be deemed refractory following repeated assessments by skilled physicians, who have obtained a rapport with the patient/ family and alongside trials of routine approaches.
- The evaluation for sedation should be made as a case conference to prevent individual physician bias or 'burnout' influencing decisions.
- If sedation is still deemed appropriate and proportionate (rarely the case), sedation should only be initiated as a temporary measure. It should be used for a pre-agreed period of respite to try to break the symptom cycle. Only after repeated trials of respite with intensive therapy should continuous sedation be considered.

The additional burden of how and when to stop treatments

The involvement of health care professionals in end-stage disease will inevitably force patients into facing explicit decisions around withholding and withdrawing treatments. As many of the treatment options will provide little or no meaningful benefit, any offer could be seen as only burdensome. Moreover the difficulty of stopping ongoing treatments such as PEG feeds, frequent blood transfusions or mechanical ventilation, even after their intended benefits have ceased, is highly charged. And the dilemma extends from patients to include their families and often draws in their health care professionals. Despite such emotive cases, arguably all patients have treatment withheld or withdrawn at some point, particularly in the hospice setting. And typically the underpinning decisions are not contentious and not always even explicit. Reassuringly, good practice means that nothing is denied to patients, as the usual mechanism will be:

- An unequivocal lack of potential efficacy
- Undisputed treatment failures
- Informed patients opting out of offered treatment
- Lack of availability, e.g. drugs not yet licensed in the UK

National consensus exists to inform decisions to withdraw or withhold life-prolonging treatment (NCHSPCS and APM, 1997b,c; BMA, 2001). It is unnecessary to duplicate this guidance. And similarly, the current legal position is readily accessible online, although it is surprisingly dynamic. While some discrepancies can be described between the professional and legal positions on withdrawing and withholding life-prolonging treatment, in the main a reassuring consensus is evident. And this guidance is gratifyingly straightforward:

- When a patient wants to continue treatment:
  - If the treatment appears to be of net benefit to that patient's health it should be offered
  - If not appearing of net benefit the treatment can be withheld or withdrawn
  - If any net benefit from the treatment is uncertain, patients should be given the offer of a trial of the treatment
- When a patient wants to stop treatment
  - Regardless of any potential benefit the treatment must be stopped

Specifically, the appropriate withdrawing treatments should not cause additional concern, realising the lack of ethical or moral distinction between an act and an omission (BMA, 2001). For example, respecting a patient's wish to turn off their ventilator should carry only the same professional burden to staff as not starting antibiotics at the end of life, even if clearly more emotive personally for the patient, family and staff (Gannon, 2005a). Ideally, stopping a futile or unwanted treatment should not add to the patient's problems, providing ongoing understanding around the treatment's purpose and mutually agreed criteria for stopping are confirmed before starting the treatment and at appropriate points during the treatment. Similarly, health care professionals need to be fully appraised of the reassuring ethical and medico-legal aspects of withdrawing treatment, and the continuity of care around explicit best interest needs to be robust. These measures should minimise the chance of crises where the patient is unprepared for making difficult decisions and feels unsupported by defensive staff, lacking in confidence.

Abuse of a privileged position

A drawback of a close professional relationship in an emotive area such as dying is that it can foster the feeling within individual staff or health care teams that they must be indispensable. Health care staff may consciously or subconsciously take on more than their training or skills allow, preventing patients from benefiting from more appropriate lines of help. For example problems can occur when health care workers feel obliged to advise on unfamiliar diseases or drugs (without adequate knowledge) or to intervene in difficult family situations, e.g. marital discord (without sufficient training). This appears particularly relevant within specialist palliative care where the 'holistic' remit seems without boundaries. Despite specialist palliative care's multidisciplinary base, continuity of care is typically provided by a single person in a single discipline (usually nursing), endeavouring to meet a vast scope of needs. An understandable but not defendable self-belief can develop, with an individual staff member or professional group seeing themselves as 'all knowledgeable' in the care of the dying. To avoid this it is necessary to improve health care workers awareness of professional and ethical boundaries, as well as providing adequate staff support and supervision in a multidisciplinary context.

Injustices in delivery of care

The delivery of health care in advanced disease will inevitably vary and risk appearing inequitable. Unfortunately real inequalities in the provision of specialist care do still occur and need to be rectified. An inconsistent availability of specialist palliative care teams fuels concerns around resource allocation, locally, nationally and internationally. There is increasing awareness of unmet needs of patients dying from non-malignant diseases and the lack of culturally sensitive services. These issues are now acknowledged as priorities to be addressed by those in palliative care (Corner and Dunlop, 1997; Doyle, 1998). Subsequently there is a conscious effort to work towards delivering high quality, appropriate 'palliative care for all' (DoH, 1998).

Globally, the medicalisation of death within 'the rich world' raises uncomfortable questions of inequity. Medical advances appear to need patients to endure increasingly toxic treatments with increasing time demands on patients, yet for seemingly only marginal increases in additional benefit, if at all. Rapidly increasing expenditure, when seeking only negligible benefits, may appear inappropriate when most in the developing world have to go without simpler, cheaper measures, which would offer far greater chances of impact (Moynihan and Smith, 2002). Rather than the pursuit of increasingly technical and expensive screening and treatment of disease, prevention would appear a worthier direction for health care to invest its time and money. In America, the top three actual causes of death appear related to tobacco, poor diet/physical inactivity and alcohol, accounting for nearly 40% of deaths (Mokdad *et al.*, 2004). As primary prevention appears the most cost-effective option, saving lives and money, medicine's obsession with diagnostic labelling and technological solutions have to be questioned (Hall, 2003).

On a national level, increased medical costs will inevitably divert resources away from other equally important areas (e.g. education, transport and crime prevention), and again the cost-effectiveness of medicine can be questioned. In particular, with charitable funding behind the vast majority of UK palliative care, by playing on the pervasive fear of a painful death, palliative care will inevitably divert attention and funding away from less emotive, less glamorous or more stigmatised, yet equally needy, areas such as mental health. Indeed, rather than parallelling patient need, increasing medicalisation may result purely from the professional or financial interests of health care providers with 'an ill for every pill' at all levels: doctors (self-interest or imperialism; to keep their jobs/status); pharmaceutical companies (greed; to boost profits); or hospice charities in the UK (self-interest; to stay afloat). The increasing acceptance of the medical model has permitted medicine to overtake patients' lives, generating escalating medical costs and a corresponding increase in medicines' ability to 'force compliance' (Hall, 2003). Conversely, health care financers, governments and insurers may wish to resist spiralling health care costs, irrespective of the potential harm to patient care (Moynihan and Smith, 2002). A 'sustainable NHS' and a health service that is 'fit for the future' are political labels in the UK that attempt to justify service cutbacks; the remaining reduced health care system will inevitably struggle to meet quality measures with an increasing focus on quantitative measures. This risks the backwards step of returning health care's focus to the biomedical model of care at the expense of the psychosocial aspects of health care; we may be left increasingly with an NHS in the UK that is only able to provide less desirable components provided by medicalisation (with increasing dependence on charitable or private funding to provide the quality aspects of medical care).

On a local level, injustices in the provision of care, whether real or perceived, may follow the further development of health care input to dying patients. Inconsistencies can be seen in the provision and delivery of specialist (and non-specialist) palliative care that occurs from one region to the next. For example, inadequacies in the approach to dying patients have been described within the hospital and community settings (Field, 1994). Corresponding inequities can be seen in specialist palliative care provision. Differences in which diagnoses qualify for input, the stage of the illness, and the range of specialist palliative care services that patients would be likely to receive can vary dramatically. And a critical review of urgent hospice admissions was left questioning the equity and appropriateness of current bed prioritisation practices (Gannon, 2005c). Even within the UK, the birthplace of the modern hospice movement, there are noticeable discrepancies in the provision of hospice beds across the country, with regional variations ranging from 34 to 65 beds per million population in 1994 (Eve et al., 1997). Additionally, the utilisation of beds did not appear consistent, such that patients may be further disadvantaged according to their geographic location. In 1995/96 the number of patients with malignant disease gaining access to hospice beds varied from 18% in Trent Region to 30% in the North West Region (NCHSPCS, 1998). Concern also surrounds hospice care's apparent 'insistence' on quality at the expense of quantity. This has led to the suggestion that 'the five star service for the select few provided by hospice organisations should be replaced by three star care for all' (Field, 1994). However, it seems puzzling that *high quality* care can now be grounds for criticism. Instead of sinking to the lowest common denominator, it would appear a more prudent objective to improve the care provided by supplying the best service to everyone who needs it; surely 'five star care for all' is the only acceptable goal. This may sound unrealistic, but independent charities are providing an add-on service to the NHS in the UK, and should not have to account for shortfalls within the NHS provision. Cost-effectiveness and rationing remain political terms for justifying suboptimal provision of care or treatments; realistically they may be necessary evils, but they cannot be championed as worthy when more than adequate national resources are arguably squandered elsewhere.

The nature of the care offered to dying patients may leave differing religious, social or cultural groups feeling neglected by a non-specific service, or worse one that appears to cater specifically for one sub-group. Hospices are criticised for catering principally for the white Christian middle classes. Indeed, in the UK 98.4% of hospice admissions are Caucasians (Eve et al., 1997), which does not reflect the country's ethnic split. There is an important cultural sensitivity that needs to be integrated into any holistic care (Tong and Spicer, 1994; Davis, 1996; McCaffrey-Boyle, 1998; Gatrad et al., 2003).

Better training for staff around awareness of cultural issues, closer integration with local communities, and sufficient resources to promote appropriate services is needed to provide greater flexibility, accessibility and acceptability of the provision of palliative care in order to reduce the apparent inequities.

Also, perhaps surprisingly, it appears that the elderly miss out on palliative care (Eve and Higginson, 2000) particularly if they have a non-cancer diagnosis (Coventry *et al.*, 2005). Dying from a non-malignant disease can present a similarly distressing picture to that seen in cancer. Patients with advanced cardiac (e.g. congestive cardiac failure), respiratory (e.g. chronic obstructive pulmonary disease), renal and liver diseases, end-stage HIV-related illnesses and progressive neurological disorders, including motor neurone disease, Parkinson's disease and dementia appear equally in need of palliative care. Unfortunately, most patients with non-malignant diseases appear greatly disadvantaged in accessing hospice services. Non-specialist palliative care provision is mandatory for all patients with advanced non-cancer illnesses, particularly once their underlying condition has become refractory to available therapies and/or the patient has made an informed decision not to pursue further active management. Complex quality of life or end-of-life issues may warrant additional specialist palliative care input at this time, just as in cancer patients. However, a disproportionately high percentage of patients with cancer receive specialist palliative care. While cancer is responsible for only a quarter of all deaths in Britain, it accounts for more than 95% of specialist palliative care workload (Eve and Higginson, 2000). This discrepancy suggests an inequity in service delivery considering the unquestionable overlaps across all terminal illnesses. Indeed, robust evidence confirms that patients with many illnesses other than cancer need hospice care. During the last year of a non-malignant illness, symptoms are prolonged and common with similar symptom prevalence to malignant illnesses (e.g. pain in about half), but sadly non-cancer patients receive less supportive care (e.g. they are less well informed by their health professionals) (Addington-Hall, 1998).

There have been many factors that have combined to give the sketchy, cancer-targeted picture of palliative care found in the UK, including:

- The original focus of the pioneers in palliative care was to improve the quality of care to end-stage cancer patients. Hospices did not set out or claim to 'tackle all the problems of terminal care' (Saunders, 1994). This founding remit has had a carry-over effect on subsequent services. However, more than forty years on, hospice services are looking ahead as how best to use the services and knowledge gained equitably.
- The resulting evidence base within palliative care has been cancer-centred, and not necessarily applicable to other diseases, just because death may be similarly close. This uncertainty has to be the prompt for more research into the symptom control of end-stage non-malignant illnesses. In the

meantime we must extrapolate as best as we can from cancer to non-cancer patients (optimally with the support of the patient's other specialists, e.g. a cardiologist in the case of heart failure).

■ The predominantly charitable nature of hospice funding has partly dictated the direction of care. The success of specific fund-raising for an emotive disease such as cancer has determined a disease-specific service, particularly in locations of high charitable donations. Increased public awareness of the needs of less high-profile diseases and more NHS funding is necessary to redress the imbalance.

■ As an evolving area of health care, 'baseline' palliative care services are still being established, leaving gaps yet to be filled. In the UK NHS measures were put in place to improve the availability of specialist palliative care (NHS Executive, 1995); these were nominally cancer orientated, even if containing demands that the benefits should extend beyond cancer patients (NHS Executive, 1996). Subsequent national development programmes have associated expansion of palliative care services directly with cancer service provision (NICE, 2004).

■ Resource limitations may reinforce discrimination; a review of health improvement plans for 1999–2003 revealed specialist palliative care, especially for non-cancer patients, was perceived as an 'optional extra' by many UK health authorities (Seymour et al., 2002).

Importantly, definitions of palliative care do not specify or suggest a cancer patient remit (NCHSPCS, 1998; WHO, 2002), despite the common misconception that palliative care is part of oncology and caters exclusively for patients with cancer. Specialist palliative care services are directed towards patients with specific indications, i.e. complex, unusual or refractory quality of life or end-of-life issues, irrespective of the patient's underlying diagnosis. The palliative approach is clearly relevant to all patients with incurable conditions (Finlay and Jones, 1995; O'Brien et al., 1998). Expert opinion, dating back nearly 15 years, has clarified that palliative care is appropriate for patients with any diagnosis causing active, progressive and advanced disease with a limited prognosis (SMAC and SNMAC, 1992). Palliative care must be delivered according to need, not by diagnosis (NHS Executive, 1996; Addington-Hall, 1998). And, research into and awareness of the palliative care needs of patients with advanced life-threatening illnesses other than cancer continues to grow (O'Brien et al., 1998; Murtagh et al., 2004; Traue and Ross, 2005; Gibbs et al., 2006; Hudson et al., 2006). Moreover, the concept of 'palliative care for all' has increasing and now near universal support (Clark, 2002); palliative care's aim to maximise the quality of life and relieve the suffering of dying patients and their families appears a basic right.

To address any imbalance in access that has disadvantaged non-cancer patients, increasingly palliative care services are openly providing 'equal access' to all patients with advanced disease, irrespective of their diagnosis. An increase of at least 79% in caseloads has been estimated if specialist palliative care services were made fully available to non-cancer patients (Addington-Hall *et al.*, 1998). Yet surprisingly, and perhaps worryingly, there hasn't been the anticipated influx of non-malignant patients. Despite the removal of barriers, non-cancer patients haven't yet been referred to specialist palliative care for assessment or advice in noticeably higher, let alone large numbers. Thus there is no evidence to support the fear that existing palliative care services would be overwhelmed by opening up to patients with non-cancer diagnoses (Kite *et al.*, 1999; Sloan, 2002). Despite such attempts to acknowledge and address any imbalance, there remains concern that non-cancer patients are still numerically under-represented within specialist palliative care activity (Addington-Hall, 1998; Addington-Hall *et al.*, 1998; Wallwork, 2000; Wasson, 2000; Ludding-ton *et al.*, 2001; Coventry *et al.*, 2005).

This mismatch, cancer seemingly being the favoured diagnosis, could merely be an appropriate reflection of the greater need/applicability of palliative care services to cancer patients. Indeed, many cancer patients also do not get input from specialist palliative care services. As many as 50% of cancer patients do not receive hospice input, as it is not needed (Eve *et al.*, 1997). And national estimates predict that only around 18% of UK cancer deaths take place in a hospice (Eve and Higginson, 2000). It is possible that the percentage of non-cancer patients requiring palliative care is lower, in part explaining the figures. However, the mismatch is more likely and more worryingly a resistance to change that spans non-cancer patients, health care professionals and society. This resistance may follow persisting historical factors (patient and professional taboos and non-thinking practices) impacting on referrals or clinical factors (uncertainties around the suitable level or timing of any palliative care input) impacting on best setting for care. But crucially, the mismatch can no longer be attributed to a blanket discrimination against non-cancer patients by palliative care services.

There are numerous clinical reasons why cancer patients may appear to need specialist care services more than other patients. However, such generalisations are always of limited value and potentially misleading. Neither cancer nor non-cancer patient groups are sufficiently uniform to allow a meaningful distinction suitable for directing guidelines, policies or services. Indeed, the majority of cancer patients receiving specialist palliative care will have significant concurrent benign pathology impacting on their symptoms and management, seemingly without problems.

With that proviso, overall, malignant diseases deliver a more predictable decline to identify an anticipatory terminal phase with a short prognosis (of 6 months or less). Ongoing specialist input for cancer patients, from oncologists, is focused on chemotherapy, radiotherapy, immunotherapy and hormone therapy against the specific underlying malignancy. As this requires the formalised use of relatively toxic treatments according to specific objective clinical measures, a clear point typically arises where 'active' oncological management will effectively stop, often many months before death. This crossroad in care results in patients having to enter more open exchanges with their lead health care professionals, unavoidably opening up discussions around the next phase of supportive care alone. The symptom picture in malignancies tends to be more variable, possibly more distressing (including more pain), and more multi-systemic, and it appears to be less predictable, with more overlapping aetiologies. Collectively this leads to the 'cancer fog' with an openly acknowledged gap in specific care provision, which necessitates the additional specific multi-professional input characteristic of specialist palliative care.

By contrast, advanced non-malignant diseases generally have a less predictable prognosis often without a clear 'terminal' phase (with more sudden deaths or prolonged survivals). Ongoing specialist input from physicians will already be more palliative and less toxic, without a clear point at which they cease to convey value. Indeed specialist physician input typically continues to have value in non-cancer diagnoses even up till the patient's death. This allows, even if counterproductive, patients to avoid confronting their disease and to distance themselves from palliative care input. Also there appears a more stable and predictable symptom picture (yet prolonged and just as important) with symptoms that can be more clearly linked to the underlying pathology, e.g. dyspnoea in heart failure (Addington-Hall, 1998). Thus ongoing specialist disease-modifying treatments (e.g. cardiology input to end-stage heart failure) may offer better symptom control for breathlessness than the more generic specialist palliative care input (particularly when realising that the palliative care evidence base and experience is skewed to cancer-related symptoms, which may or may not be applicable). Regardless, at this stage all medical care should still be informed by palliative care principles, adding in specialist palliative care when particularly complex problems are encountered (Addington-Hall, 1998) even if this care provision will need modification (Traue and Ross, 2005); possibly requiring differing pharmacological approaches, greater monitoring and enduring collaborative inter-specialty practice.

Rightly or wrongly, it is possible that a disproportionate number of cancer patients will still need, or inevitably continue to get, specialist palliative care input compared with non-cancer patients. To safeguard equitable practices, the priorities are: clarifying (to both professionals and public) that access is determined by specialist need and not diagnosis; to consider every case on an individual basis; and to check the appropriateness of delivery of care to all patients (to ensure that it is not unfairly biased towards any subgroup).

Five barriers restricting increases in palliative care to non-cancer patients have be described: current skills within specialist palliative care, difficulties in discriminating appropriate patients, acceptability within potential patients, additional resource implications, and the vested interests of present health care provision (Field and Addington-Hall, 1999). Work continues to address these issues. Validated prognostic models to provide objective measures of palliative status and evaluation of specialist palliative care input to non-cancer patients are needed (Wallwork, 2000; Luddington *et al.*, 2001; Coventry *et al.*, 2005). Already, work has recently described variations in illness trajectory according to diagnosis, and explored how this may affect provision of palliative care (Murtagh *et al.*, 2004). Improving assess to palliative care for patients with non-cancer diagnoses should also be helped by national initiatives in the UK introducing National Service Frameworks which stipulate the need for palliative care in conditions such as coronary heart disease, renal disease and long-term neurological conditions (Traue and Ross, 2005).

Concluding thoughts

The term 'medicalisation of death' was originally coined to describe the secular and institutionalised attitudes to death of 'modern' society. Despite many possible interpretations its use now conveys a negative connotation of 'over-medicalisation'. As the medical care available to patients with terminal illness increases it appears just as unhelpful to label all medical input as wrong, as it is unhelpful to pretend that medicine has the answer for all ills or comes without drawbacks. The priority is to review how much medical input should be provided... the right amount, in the right way, at the right time, for the right people.

An enduring right of access to the best available health care is central to a caring society. Within this, the discipline of medicine sets out to relieve suffering as well as cure disease. By the time a patient has an advanced disease that has progressed beyond cure, the focus of medical input will shift to centre on the relief of any suffering. Though somewhat at odds with the current biomedical view of medicine, the value of this medical input in caring for the terminally ill could not be more relevant, delivering benefits in both quantitative survival and quality of remaining life. Allowing for the contrasts in different patients' needs and the scope of health care available there appears merit in offering a tailored medical input to the care of the dying. A thorough medical assessment is required to identify or exclude the need for medical input (at that time), and to provide the patient with the necessary information (if desired) to make informed decisions and thus have true autonomy. Though the palpable medical role may be limited in many cases, there will remain a significant role for medicine in supporting the input from different professional groups. However, dying patients do not need a compulsory medical input, just its consideration and availability when an agreed and achievable benefit can be identified. Medicine does not claim an extraordinary jurisdiction over dying people, nor can it singularly offer a better death; but neither can it be absent (Holstein, 1997).

Unfortunately, medical input at the end of life comes at a cost: both the potential for causing harm to patients and their families, and to undermine other professional groups and divert resources from equally deserving areas. Numerous drawbacks can be identified in the present delivery of medical care to the terminally ill. However, rather than prompting the rejection of medicine and all it offers, these concerns should serve as the necessary spur to improve the quality of medical input to the dying. The future lies in continued education of the health care community to better understand the value of care (rather than just cure), and to transform the death of a patient back onto a human scale. This will need an increased awareness and integration of medical ethics into everyday practice. Ethics can secure the quality of care; for example, by formulating the necessary condemnation of futile or burdensome therapies offered only to be doing *everything* possible, rather than doing the right thing (Escalante *et al.*, 1997). Alongside this, public and patient education to clarify patients' rights, to foster realistic and balanced expectations of medicine (the good and the bad bits) and to facilitate coping mechanisms to reduce unnecessary overdependence on health care professionals is needed.

Similarly, nursing and other professions, such as physical therapies and social work, are ideally positioned to have a dramatic impact on patients by considering health care issues within the context of a person's activities of daily living. This attention to individual functioning further refines quality of life issues to complement other provided care. Quality of life becomes the key goal as death approaches, and the distinctions between the different health care professionals' roles and non-health care interventions inevitably blur. This overlap should be seen as an opportunity for flexibility to provide more extensive and appropriate benefits to patients as death approaches.

Members of modern societies find the naturalness of death and dying hard to accept (Field, 1994). This avoidance by society of the inevitability of death appears to be a coping mechanism for which medicine cannot be held accountable. Medicine may offer life-prolonging treatment, and though death may be postponed, it can never be evaded. Life-prolonging treatment is not restricted to the care of the dying, but an everyday occurrence in medicine. Even simple infections could be fatal without appropriate antibiotic treatment. And this applies equally to patients with far-advanced disease. Thus the question is not whether the pursuit of life-prolonging treatment is right or wrong in the care of terminally ill patients, but whether it is acceptable or unacceptable to the patient. Medicine retains a legal and moral duty to offer treatments that are in the patient's best interests. This responsibility for deciding appropriate health care is a clinical issue that cannot adequately be abdicated to others. However, whether to accept offered treatments remains the decision of the patient alone. It is not for relatives, physicians, nurses or society to impose their value system on an individual simply because they have become terminally ill. A person's worth and basic rights are not lessened in any way by an advancing disease.

As each person is unique, so is his or her death. It is an exclusively personal state, and though parts may be shared, as bystanders we are unlikely to see more than a glimpse of the true picture, each of us from a different perspective. The patient experience is based on their disease, their personality, and the available support, in the context of prior life events, in particular any dealings with death. Their perceptions will be constantly changing, as each new moment will generate new issues. There will also be additional external influences from society and a patient's cultural background. Consequently, each dying patient's requirements will be unique, though these will be likely to include some degree of medical input at some time. This medical need should never be presumed or denied out of hand, but assessed and delivered when required as part of the 'total care' of patients with terminal illnesses. This should ensure that any 'medicalisation of death' could be seen as a valued component of care. Just as medicine should not dictate the path of dying, philosophers and sociologists should not expect to impose their belief systems to turn terminal patients away from the benefits of medicine. Instead, a collaborative approach would seem to be in our patients' and society's best interests (McCue, 1995). This is the ideal embodied in specialist palliative care's multidisciplinary approach, which looks to all avenues for guidance in how to deliver the best care to dying patients.

Specialist palliative care integrates medicine, nursing, social work, pastoral/spiritual care, physiotherapy, occupational therapy, pharmacy and other related disciplines. The availability of specialist palliative care is well established as a prerequisite component of cancer care in the UK (Calman and Hine, 1995; NICE, 2004). And there is increasing support for this input to be available to all far-advanced diseases. The blend of disciplines allows palliative care to provide a holistic approach for those with an identifiable need who request it. Though medical input provides a significant component of this care, the term 'medicalisation' appears to undervalue such a broad mix of skills that combines to deliver patient-centred support incorporating physical, emotional, spiritual, and social elements. Palliative care is expanding rapidly, with increasing expectations from specialist and non-specialist health care to dying patients. Although this input cannot escape the label 'medicalisation', it may with time evoke a more positive use of the term.

Unfortunately, theory and practice do not always meet, and many problems are acknowledged within palliative care provision. This is not surprising considering the emotive mix of complex clinical, social and ethical dilemmas within care of the dying and the high resource implications that follow. However, they remain key areas to address within palliative care, which constantly aims to improve the quality of care provided to dying patients. Despite the actual and potential problems, the proven benefit from palliative care interventions generates overwhelming support for health care involvement in the care of the dying on a pragmatic basis.

There are no generalisations possible in dealing with death and dying. The value of philosophical, sociological, spiritual and medical/nursing models of death lies in aiding research and academic understanding. However, it would be a mistake to hide behind such banners and claim that the existing care of the dying is good or bad according to any one system. Any single-mindedness may divert possible support from the attentiveness and loving relationships central to life's end (Holstein, 1997). It is easy to criticise the existing health care model of input to dying patients. However, no 'system' will ever do justice to the complex, dynamic, intensive, numerous, and at times irresolute needs of the terminally ill. Thus we must resist falling in with the criticisms of health care interventions that are freely voiced without proposing much in the way of practical alternatives. It would be unwise to repeat the mistakes of the past and return to a nihilistic state, undoing all the progress that has already been made. We must all humble ourselves, and acknowledge that dying is not always open to solutions (Holstein, 1997). Equally we must endeavour to do what we can and not abandon people as their death approaches.

References

The following references are for both Chapter 4 and Chapter 5.

Addington-Hall, J. (1998) (for Working Party of The National Council for Hospices and Specialist Palliative Care Services (NCHSPCS) and The Scottish Partnership Agency (SPA) (1998) Reaching out: specialist palliative care for adults with non-malignant diseases. *Occasional Paper 14*. London.

Addington-Hall, J. and McCarthy, M. (1995) Dying from cancer: results of a national population based investigation. *Palliative Medicine*, 9, 295–305.

Addington-Hall, J., Fakhoury, W. and McCarthy, M. (1998) Specialist palliative care in nonmalignant disease. *Palliative Medicine*, 12(6), 417–27.

Ahmedzai, S. (1997) Five years five threads (Editorial). *Progress in Palliative Care*, 5, 235–7.

Airedale NHS Trust v Bland (1993) Airedale NHS Trust v Bland [1993] 1 All ER 821.

Archer, V. R., Billingham, L. J. and Cullen, M. H. (1999) Palliative chemotherapy: no longer a contradiction in terms. *The Oncologist*, 4, 470–7.

Ashby, M. (1998) Palliative care, death causation, public policy and the law. *Progress in Palliative Care*, 6(3), 69–77.

Ashby, M. and Stoffel, B. (1991) Therapeutic ratio and defined phases: proposal of ethical framework for palliative care. *British Medical Journal*, 302, 1322–4.

Barclay, S. I. G., Todd, C. J., Grade, G. E. and Lipscombe, J. (1997) How common is medical training in palliative care? A postal survey of General Practitioners. *British Journal of General Practice*, **47**, 800–5.

Beauchamp, T. and Childress, J. (1994) *The Principles of Biomedical Ethics*, 4th edn. Oxford University Press, Oxford.

Bevan, D. (1998) Death, dying and inequality. *Care – The Journal of Practice and Development*, **7**(1), 27–38.

Boyd, K. (2001) Deciding about resuscitation. *Journal of Medical Ethics*, **27**, 291–4.

Bradshaw, A. (1996) The spiritual dimension of hospice: the secularization of an ideal. *Social Science and Medicine*, **43**(3), 409–19.

British Medical Association (BMA) (2001) *Withholding and Withdrawing Life-prolonging Medical Treatment. Guidance for Decision-making*, 2nd edn. BMJ Books, London.

British Medical Association (BMA), the Resuscitation Council (UK) and Royal College of Nursing (RCN) (2002) *Decisions Relating to Cardiopulmonary Resuscitation: a Joint Statement*. Available on-line at http://www.bma.org.uk/ap.nsf/AttachmentsByTitle/PDFcardioresus/$FILE/Cardio.pdf (accessed 9 November 2006).

Buckman, R. (1996) Talking to patients about cancer. *British Medical Journal*, **313**, 699–700.

Calman, K. (1992) *Annual report for 1990/1991 Resuscitation Policy*, PL/CMO (91) 22.26. Chief Medical Officer/Health Service Commissioner, London.

Calman, K. and Hine, D. (On behalf of the expert advisory group on cancer to the chief medical officers) (1995) *A Policy Framework for Commissioning Cancer Services"* Department of Health/Welsh Office, London.

Cherney, N. I. (1998) Commentary: sedation in response to refractory existential distress: walking the fine line. *Journal of Pain and Symptom Management*, **16**(6), 404–6.

Clark, D. (2002) Between hope and acceptance: the medicalisation of dying. *British Medical Journal*, **324**, 905–7.

Clark, D. and Seymour, J. (1999) Routinisation and medicalisation. In: *Reflections on Palliative Care*, pp. 104–24. Open University Press, Buckingham.

Clark, J. (2003) Patient centred death. *British Medical Journal*, **327**, 174–5.

Clover, A. and Kassab, S. (1998) Complementary medicine for patients with cancer. *European Journal of Palliative Care*, **5**(3), 73–6.

Conill, C., Verger, E., Henriquez, I., Saiz, N., Espier, M., Lugo, F. and Garrigos, A. (1997) Symptom prevalence in the last week of life. *Journal of Pain and Symptom Management*, **14**(6), 328–31.

Corner, J. (1997) More openness needed in palliative care. *British Medical Journal*, **315**, 1242.

Corner, J. and Dunlop, R. (1997) New approaches to care. In: *New Themes in Palliative Care* (eds. D. Clark, J. Hochley and S. Ahmedzai). Open University Press, Buckingham.

Costantini, M., Higginson, I. J., Boni, L., Orengo, M. A., Garrone, E., Henriquet, F. and Bruzzi, P. (2003) Effect of a palliative home care team on hospital admissions among patients with advanced cancer. *Palliative Medicine*, **17**(4), 315–21.

Coventry, P. A., Grande, G. E., Richards, D. A. and Todd, C. J. (2005) Prediction of appropriate timing of palliative care for older adults with non-malignant life-threatening disease: a systematic review. *Age and Ageing*, **34**(3), 218–27.

Craig, G. M. (1994) On withholding nutrition and hydration in the terminally ill: has palliative medicine gone too far? *Journal of Medical Ethics*, **20**, 139–43.

Craig, G. M. (1996) On withholding artificial hydration and nutrition from terminally ill sedated patients. The debate continues. *Journal of Medical Ethics*, **22**(3), 147–53.

Davis, A. (1996) Ethics and ethnicity: end-of-life decisions in four ethnic groups of cancer patients. *Medicine and Law*, **15**(3), 429–32.

Department of Health (DoH) (1998) *Palliative Care*. Health Service Circular HSC 1998/115. Department of Health, Wetherby.

Department of Health (DoH) (2004) *Manual for Cancer Services*. NHS Crown Copyright.

dictionary.com (2006) http://dictionary.reference.com/ (accessed 15 August 2006).

Donelly, S. (1999) Folklore associated with dying in the west of Ireland. *Palliative Medicine*, **13**, 57–62.

Doyle, D. (1998) Domiciliary palliative care. In: *Oxford Textbook of Palliative Medicine*, 2nd edn (eds. D. Doyle, G. Hanks and N. MacDonald), pp. 657–953. Oxford University Press, New York.

Dunlop, R. J., Ellershaw, J. E., Baines, M. J., Sykes, N. and Saunders, C. M. (1995) On withholding artificial hydration and nutrition in the terminally ill; has palliative medicine gone too far? *Journal of Medical Ethics*, **21**(3), 141–3.

Dunphy, K. and Randall, F. (1997) Ethical decision-making in palliative care. *European Journal of Palliative Care*, **4**(4), 126–8.

Dunphy, K., Finlay, I., Rathbone, G., Gilbert, J. and Hicks, F. (1995) Rehydration in palliative and terminal care: if not why not? *Palliative Medicine*, **9**, 221–8.

Ellershaw, J. E. (2002) Clinical pathways for care of the dying – an innovation to disseminate clinical excellence. *Journal of Palliative Medicine*, **5**(4), 617–23.

Ellershaw, J. E. and Ward, C. (2003) Care of the dying patient: the last hours or days of life. *British Medical Journal*, **326**, 30–4.

Ellershaw, J. E., Peat, S. J. and Boys, L. C. (1995) Assessing the effectiveness of a hospital palliative care team. *Palliative Medicine*, **9**(2), 145–52.

Escalante, C. P., Martin, C. G., Elting, L. S. R. and Rubenstein, E. B. (1997) Medical futility and appropriate medical care in patients whose death is thought to be imminent. *Supportive Care in Cancer*, **5**(4), 274–80.

Eve, A. and Higginson, I. J. (2000) Minimum dataset activity for hospice and hospital palliative care services in the UK 1997/98. *Palliative Medicine*, **14**(5), 395–404.

Eve, A., Smith, A. M. and Tebbit, P. (1997) Hospice and palliative care trends in the UK 1994–5, including a summary of trends 1990–5. *Palliative Medicine*, **11**, 31–43.

Fainsinger, R. L., Waller, A., Bercovici, M., Bengtson, K., Landman, W., Hosking, M., Nunez-Olarte, J. and deMoissac, D. (2000) A multicentre international study of sedation for uncontrolled symptoms in terminally ill patients. *Palliative Medicine*, **14**(4), 257–65.

Farsides, C. C. S. (1998) Autonomy and its implications for palliative care: a northern European perspective. *Palliative Medicine*, **12**(3), 147–51.

Feuer, D. (1998) Organ donation in palliative care. *European Journal of Palliative Care*, **5**(1), 21–5.

Field, D. (1994) Palliative medicine and the medicalization of death. *European Journal of Cancer Care*, **3**, 58–62.

Field, D. and Addington-Hall, J. (1999) Extending specialist palliative care to all? *Social Science and Medicine*, **48**(9), 1271–80.

Finlay, I. G. and Jones, R. V. H. (1995) Definitions in palliative care (letter). *British Medical Journal*, **311**, 754.

Forbes, K. and Huxtable, R. (2006) Clarifying the data on double effect (editorial). *Palliative Medicine*, **20**, 395–6.

Fordham, S., Dowrick, C. and May, C. (1998) Palliative medicine: is it really specialist territory? *Journal of the Royal Society of Medicine*, **91**, 568–72.

Gannon, C. (1995) Cancer patients' place of death (letter). *British Journal of General Practice*, **45**(400), 630.

Gannon, C. (2004a) Voluntary refusal of food and fluids: a personal view from the UK. *International Journal of Palliative Nursing*, **10**(5), 242–3.

Gannon, C. (2004b) Reflections on clinical audit in palliative care following an attempt to audit urinary catheterization. *International Journal of Palliative Nursing*, **10**(11), 524–32.

Gannon, C. (2005a) A request for hospice admission from hospital to withdraw ventilation. *The Journal of Medical Ethics*, **31**(7), 383–4.

Gannon, C. (2005b) Will the lead clinician please stand up? *British Medical Journal*, **330**, 737.

Gannon, C. (2005c) Hidden aspects in urgent hospice admissions. In: *Hidden Aspects in Palliative Care* (eds. B. Nyatanga and M. Astley-Pepper). Quay, London.

Garwin, M. (1998) The duty to care – the right to refuse. *The Journal of Legal Medicine*, **19**, 99–125.

Gatrad, A. R., Brown, E., Notta, H. and Sheikh, A. (2003) Palliative care needs of minorities. *British Medical Journal*, **327**, 176–7.

Gaze, M. N., Kelly, C. G., Kerr, G. R., Cull, A., Cowie, V. J., Gregor, A., Howard, G. C. W. and Rodger, A. (1997) Pain relief and quality of life following radiotherapy for bone metastases a randomised trail of two fractionation schedules. *Radiotherapy and Oncology*, **45**, 109–16.

General Medical Council (1998) *Maintaining Good Medical Practice*. General Medical Council, London.

George, R. J. D., Finlay, I. G. and Jeffrey, D. (2005) Legalised euthanasia will violate the rights of vulnerable patients. *British Medical Journal*, **331**, 684–5.

Gibbs, L. M. E., Khatri, A. K. and Gibbs, S. R. (2006) Survey of specialist palliative care and heart failure: September 2004. *Palliative Medicine*, **20**, 603–9.

Grande, G. E., Barclay, S. I. G. and Todd, C. J. (1997) Difficulty of symptom control and General Practitioners' knowledge of patients' symptoms. *Palliative Medicine*, **11**, 399–406.

Grande, G. E., Todd, C. J., Barclay, S. I. G. and Farquhar, M. C. (1999) Does hospital at home for palliative care facilitate death at home? Randomised controlled trial. *British Medical Journal*, **319**, 1472–75.

Griffiths, A. and Beaver, K. (1997) Quality of life during high dose chemotherapy for breast cancer. *International Journal of Palliative Nursing*, **3**(3), 138–44.

Hall, B. A. (2003) An essay on an authentic meaning of medicalization. The patient's perspective. *Advances in Nursing Science*, **26**(1), 53–62.

Hanson, L. C., Danis, M. and Garret, J. (1997) What is wrong with end-of-life care? Opinions of bereaved family members. *Journal of the American Geriatrics Society*, **45**(11), 1339–44.

Hardy, J. (1996) Endocrine therapy in advanced malignancy. *European Journal of Palliative Care*, **2**(4), 151–4.

Her Majesty's Stationery Office (HMSO) (2004) Human Tissue Act 2004 Chapter 30, Queen's Printer of Acts of Parliament. Available online at http://www.opsi.gov.uk/acts/acts2004/20040030.htm (accessed 2 September 2006).

Her Majesty's Stationery Office (HMSO) (2005) Mental Capacity Act 2005 Chapter 9, Queen's Printer of Acts of Parliament. Available online at http://www.opsi.gov.uk/acts/acts2005/20050009.htm (accessed 22 August 2006).

Higginson, I. J. (1998) Who needs palliative care? (editorial). *Journal of the Royal Society of Medicine*, **91**(11), 563–4.

Higginson, I. J., Astin, P. and Dolan, S. (1998) Where do cancer patients die? Ten year trends in the place of death of cancer patients in England. *Palliative Medicine*, **12**, 353–63.

Hinton, J. (1994a) Can home care maintain an acceptable quality of life for patients with terminal cancer and their relatives? *Palliative Medicine*, **8**(3), 183–96.

Hinton, J. (1994b) Which patients with terminal cancer are admitted from home care? *Palliative Medicine*, **8**(3), 197–210.

Holstein, M. (1997) Reflections on death and dying. *Academic Medicine*, **72**(10), 848–55.

Hospice Information Service (2006) *Directory of Hospice and Palliative Care Services in the United Kingdom and Ireland*. St Christopher's, London.

Hoy, A. (1999) Routinisation and medicalisation. *European Journal of Palliative Care*, **6**(6), 178.

Hudson, P. L., Toye, C. and Kristjanson, L. J. (2006) Would people with Parkinson's disease benefit from palliative care? *Palliative Medicine*, **20**, 87–94.

Hunt, R. (1997) Place of death of cancer patients; choice versus constraint. *Progress in Palliative Care*, **5**(6), 238–42.

Illich, I. (1990) *Limits to Medicine: Medical Nemesis: the Expropriation of Health*. Penguin, London.

Jack, B., Hillier, V., Williams, A. and Oldham, J. (2003) Hospital-based palliative care teams improve the symptoms of cancer patients. *Palliative Medicine*, **17**(6), 498–502.

Jeffery, P. and Millard, P. H. (1997) An ethical framework for clinical decision-making at the end of life. *Journal of the Royal Society of Medicine*, **90**, 504–6.

Johnson, I. S., Rogers, C., Biswas, B. and Admedzai, S. (1990) What do hospices do? *British Medical Journal*, **300**, 791–3.

Jordhoy, M. S. and Grande, G. (2006) Living alone and dying at home: a realistic alternative? *European Journal of Palliative Care*, **13**(6), 244–7.

Kite, S., Jones, K. and Tookman, A. (1999) Specialist palliative care and patients with noncancer diagnoses; the experience of a service. *Palliative Medicine*, **13**(6), 477–84.

Kite, S. M., Maher, E. J., Anderson, K., Young, T., Young, J., Wood, J., Howells, N. and Bradburn, J. (1998) Development of an aromatherapy service at a cancer centre. *Palliative Medicine*, **12**, 171–80.

Lam, P., Chan, K., Tse, C. and Leung, M. (2005) Retrospective analysis of antibiotic use and survival in advanced cancer patients with infections. *Journal of Pain and Symptom Management*, **30**(6), 536–43.

Lapum, J. L. (2003) In search of a good death: a good death and medicalisation need not be polarised. *British Medical Journal*, **327**, 224–5.

Latimer, E. (1991) Caring for seriously ill and dying patients: the philosophy and ethics. *Canadian Medical Association Journal*, **144**(7), 859–64.

Luddington, L., Cox, S., Higginson, I. and Livesley, B. (2001) The need for palliative care for patients with non-cancer diseases: a review of the evidence. *International Journal of Palliative Nursing*, **7**(5), 221–6.

Macleod, R. and Schumacher, M. (1999) Hospice management – translating the vision. *European Journal of Palliative Care*, **6**(6), 194–7.

Maddocks, I. (1998a) Change and progress (editorial). *Progress in Palliative Care*, **6**(1), 1–3.

Maddocks, I. (1998b) Explaining palliative care – to the law and to others (editorial). *Progress in Palliative Care*, **6**(3), 67–8.

Maiwand, M. O. (1998) Cryotherapy for management of endobronchial obstruction. *CME Bulletin Palliative Medicine*, **1**(1), 16–20.

Mason, J. K. and McCall Smith, R. A. (1991) *Law and Medical Ethics*, 3rd edn, p. 402. Butterworth, London.

McCaffrey-Boyle, D. (1998) The cultural context of dying from cancer. *International Journal of Palliative Nursing*, **4**(2), 709–83.

McCue, J. D. (1995) The naturalness of dying. *Journal of the American Medical Association*, **273**(13), 1039–43.

McNamara, B., Waddell, C. and Colvin, M. (1994) The institutionalization of the good death. *Social Science and Medicine*, **39**(11), 1501–8.

McNamara, B., Waddell, C. and Colvin, M. (1995) Threats to the good death: the cultural context of stress and coping among hospice nurses. *Sociology of Health and Illness*, **17**(2), 222–44.

Meystre, C. J. N., Burley, N. M. J. and Ahmedzai, S. (1997) What investigations and procedures do patients in hospices want? Interview based survey of patients and their nurses. *British Medical Journal*, **315**, 1202–3.

Middleton, G. W., Smith, I. E., O'Brien, M. E. R., Norton, A., Hickish, T., Priest, K., Spencer, L. and Ashley, S. (1998) Good symptom relief with palliative MVP (Mitomycin-C, Vinblastine and Cisplatin) chemotherapy in malignant mesothelioma. *Annals of Oncology*, **9**, 269–73.

Moe, C. and Schroll, M. (1998) Choice of treatment among residents of nursing homes in case of life threatening disease (English summary) *Ugeskr Laeger*, **26**, 160(5), 638–43.

Mokdad, A. H., Marks, J. S., Stroup, D. F. and Gerberding, J. L. (2004) Actual causes of death in the United States, 2000. *Journal of the American Medical Association*, **291**, 1238–45.

Morrison, R. S. and Morris, J. (1995) When there is no cure: palliative care for the dying patient. *Geriatrics*, **50**(7), 45–51.

Moynihan, R. and Smith, R. (2002) Too much medicine? *British Medical Journal*, **324**, 859–60.

Murtagh, F. E., Preston, M. and Higginson, I. (2004) Patterns of dying: palliative care for non-malignant disease. *Clinical Medicine*, **4**(1), 39–44.

National Council for Hospice and Specialist Palliative Care Services (NCHSPCS) (1995) *Specialist Palliative Care: A Statement of Definitions*. Occasional Paper 8. National Council for Hospice and Specialist Palliative Services, London.

National Council for Hospice and Specialist Palliative Care Services (NCHSPCS) (1998) *A Guide to the Commissioning of Palliative Care Services for Adults*. National Council for Hospice and Specialist Palliative Services, London.

National Council for Hospice and Specialist Palliative Care Services (NCHSPCS) and the Association for Palliative Medicine of Great Britain and Ireland (APM) (1997a) *Voluntary Euthanasia: The Council's View*. National Council for Hospice and Specialist Palliative Services, London.

National Council for Hospices and Specialist Palliative Care Services (NCHSPCS) and the Association for Palliative Medicine of Great Britain and Ireland (APM) Joint Working Party (1997b) CPR for people who are terminally ill. *European Journal of Palliative Care*, **4**(4), 125.

National Council for Hospices and Specialist Palliative Care Services of (NCHSPCS) and the Association for Palliative Medicine of Great Britain and Ireland (APM) Joint Working Party (1997c) Artificial hydration (AH) for people who are terminally ill. *European Journal of Palliative Care*, **4**(4), 124.

National Health Service (NHS) Executive (1995) *Cover for The Expert Advisory Group on cancer to the Chief Medical Officers of England and Wales. A Policy Framework for Commissioning Cancer Services*, EL(95) 51. NHS Executive, London.

National Health Service (NHS) Executive (1996) *A Policy Framework for Commissioning Cancer Services: Palliative Care Services*, EL (96) 85. NHS Executive, London.

National Institute for Clinical Excellence (NICE) (2004) *Improving Supportive and Palliative Care for Adults with Cancer*. National Institute for Clinical Excellence, London.

Noble, S., Hargreaves, P. and Dingwall, A. (2000) Successful cardiopulmonary resuscitation in a hospice. *Palliative Medicine*, **15**(4), 440–1.

O'Brien, T., Welsh, J. and Dunn, F. G. (1998) ABC of palliative care. Non-malignant conditions. *British Medical Journal*, **316**(7127), 286–9.

Palmer, C., Higginson, I. and Jones, P. (1998) Hospice at home (letter). *British Journal of General Practice*, **48**, 1006.

Patchell, R. A., Tibbs, P. A., Regine, W. F., Payne, R., Saris, S., Kryscio, R. J., Mohiuddin, M. and Young, B. (2005) Direct decompressive surgical resection in the treatment of spinal cord compression caused by metastatic cancer: a randomised trial. *Lancet*, **366**(9486), 643–8.

Payne, S. A., Langley-Evans, A. and Hillier, R. (1996) Perceptions of a good death: comparative study of the views of hospice staff and patients. *Palliative Medicine*, **10**, 307–12.

R (Burke) v GMC (2005) R (on the application of Burke) v GMC [2005] EWCA Civ 1003.

Re B (2002) Re B (Consent to treatment: capacity) [2002] All ER 449.

Re (Burke) v GMC (2004) Re (Burke) v The General Medical Council [2004] EWHC 1879 (Admin).

Re C (1994) Re C (Adult Refusal of Treatment) [1994] 1 WLR 290.

Rogers, R v Swindon NHS Primary Care Trust (2006) Rogers, R (on the application of) v Swindon NHS Primary Care Trust and Secretary of State for Health [2006] EWHC 171 (Admin) (15 February 2006).

Rogue, D., Temon, N., Albarede, J. and Arbus, L. (1994) Questions raised by artificial prolongation of life in the aged patient. *Medicine and Law*, **13**, 269–375.

Rowell, N. P. and Gleeson, F. V. (2002) Steroids, radiotherapy, chemotherapy and stents for superior vena caval obstruction in carcinoma of the bronchus: a systemic review. *Clinical Oncology*, **14**, 338–51.

Samanta, A. and Samanta, J. (2006) Advance directives, best interests and clinical judgement: shifting sands at the end of life. *Clinical Medicine, Journal of the Royal College of Physicians*, **6**(3), 274–8.

Saunders, C. (1994) (Letter) *European Journal of Cancer Care*, **4**, 148.

Saunders, C. (1998) Caring for cancer. *Journal of the Royal Society of Medicine*, **91**, 439–441.

Scally, G. and Donaldson, L. J. (1998) Looking forward: clinical governance and the drive for quality improvement in the new NHS in England. *British Medical Journal*, **317**, 61–5.

Seale, C., Addington-Hall, J. and McCarthy, M. (1997) Awareness of dying: prevalence, causes and consequences. *Social Science and Medicine*, **45**(3), 477–84.

Seamark, D. A., Thorne, C. P., Lawrence, C. and Gray, D. J. (1995) Appropriate place of death for cancer patients; views of General Practitioners and hospital doctors. *British Journal of General Practice*, **45**(396), 359–63.

Seymour, J., Clark, D. and Marples, R. (2002) Palliative care and policy in England: a review of health improvement plans for 1999–2003. *Palliative Medicine*, **16**(1), 5–11.

Shaiova, L. (1998) Case presentation: 'terminal sedation' and existential distress. *Journal of Pain and Symptom Management*, **16**(6), 403–4.

Silvestri, G., Pritchard, R. and Welch, H. G. (1998) Preferences for chemotherapy in patients with advanced non-small cell lung cancer: descriptive study based on scripted interviews. *British Medical Journal*, **317**, 771–5.

Slevin, M. L., Plant, L., Wilson, H. J., Wilson, P., Gregory, W. M., Armes, P. J. and Downer, S. M. (1990) Attitudes to chemotherapy; comparing views of patients with cancer with those of doctors, nurses and general public. *British Medical Journal*, **300**, 1458–60.

Sloan, R. H. (2002) Palliative care can be useful in cardiovascular disease. *British Medical Journal*, **324**, 1035.

Standing Medical Advisory Committee and Standing Nurse and Midwifery Advisory Committee (SMAC and SNMAC) (1992) *The Principles and Provision of Palliative Care*. Joint report of the Standing Medical Advisory Committee and Standing Nurse and Midwifery Advisory Committee. HMSO, London.

Stanley, J. M. (1992) The Appleton International Conference: developing guidelines for decisions to forego life-prolonging medical treatment. *Journal of Medical Ethics*, **18**(sup), 3–5.

Stationery Office, The (TSO) (1983) Mental Health Act 1983. The Stationery Office, London.

Swanson, J. W. and McCrary, S. V. (1996) Medical futility decisions and physicians' legal defensiveness: the impact of anticipated conflicts on thresholds for end-of-life treatment. *Social Science and Medicine*, **42**(1), 125–32.

Sykes, N. and Thorns, A. (2003a) Sedative use in the last week of life and the implications for end-of-life decision making. *Archives of Internal Medicine*, **163**, 341–44.

Sykes, N. and Thorns, A. (2003b) The use of opioids and sedatives at the end of life. *Lancet Oncology*, **4**(5), 312–18.

Sze, W. M., Shelley, M. D., Held, I., Wilt, T. J. and Mason, M. D. (2003) Palliation of metastatic bone pain: single fraction versus multifraction radiotherapy – a systematic review of randomised trials. *Clinical Oncology (Royal College Radiologists)*, **15**(6), 345–52.

Tebbit, P. (2006) Personal communication, September 2006; Payment by results presentation, The Princess Alice Hospice, Esher, Surrey, UK.

Thatcher, N., Anderson, H., Betticher, D. C. and Ranson, M. (1995) Symptomatic benefit from gemcitabine and other chemotherapy in advanced non-small cell lung cancer: changes in performance status and tumour related symptoms. *Anti-Cancer Drugs*, **6**(sup 6), 39–48.

Thomas, C., Morris, S. M. and Clark, D. (2004) Place of death: preferences among cancer patients and their carers. *Social Science and Medicine*, **58**(12), 2431–44.

Thorns, A. (1998a) Doctrine of double effect means that death is not intended (letter). *British Medical Journal*, **316**, 391.

Thorns, A. (1998b) A review of the doctrine of double effect. *European Journal of Palliative Care*, **5**(4), 117–20.

Thorns, A. R. and Ellershaw, J. E. (1999) A survey of nursing and medical staff views on the use of cardiopulmonary resuscitation in the hospice. *Palliative Medicine*, **13**, 225–32.

Tong, K. L. and Spicer, B. J. (1994) The Chinese palliative patient and family in North America: a cultural perspective. *Journal of Palliative Care*, **10**(1), 26–8.

Traue, D. C. and Ross, J. R. (2005) Palliative care in non-malignant diseases. *Journal of the Royal Society of Medicine*, **98**, 503–6.

Twycross, R. (1997) *Symptom Management in Advanced Cancer*, 2nd edn. Radcliffe Medical Press, Oxford.

Twycross, R., Wilcock, A., Charlesworth, S. and Dickman, A. (2002) *PCF2: Palliative Care Formulary*, 2nd edn. Radcliffe Medical Press, Oxford.

Vainio, A. and Auvinen, A. with Members of the Symptom Prevalence Group (1996) Prevalence of symptoms among patients with advanced cancer: an international collaborative study. *Journal of Pain and Symptom Management*, **12**(1), 3–10.

Wallwork, L. (2000) Palliative care in non-malignant disease: a pragmatic response. *International Journal of Palliative Nursing*, **6**(4), 186–91.

Wasson, K. (2000) Ethical arguments for providing palliative care to non-cancer patients. *International Journal of Palliative Nursing*, **6**(2), 66–70.

Watson, M. S., Lucas, C. F., Hoy, A. M. and Back, I. N. (2005) *Oxford Handbook of Palliative Care*. Oxford University Press, Oxford.

White, K. (1999) Increased medicalization within palliative care. *International Journal of Palliative Nursing*, **5**(3), 108–9.

World Health Organization (WHO) (1958) *The First Ten Years. The World Health Organization*. WHO, Geneva.

World Health Organization (WHO) (1990) *Cancer Pain Relief and Palliative Care: Report of a WHO Expert Committee*. WHO, Geneva.

World Health Organization (WHO) (2002) *WHO Definition of Palliative Care*. WHO, Geneva. Available online at http://www.who.int/cancer/palliative/definition/en/ (accessed 19 August 2006).

Wu, J. S. Y., Monk, G., Clark, T., Robinson, J., Eigl, B. J. C. and Hagen, N. (2006) Palliative radiotherapy improves pain and reduces functional interference in patients with painful bone metastases: a quality assurance study. *Clinical Oncology*, **18**, 539–44.

CHAPTER 6

Ethical issues surrounding death and dying

Simon Chippendale

Death does not frighten me; it is the jump I am afraid of (Simone de Beauvoir, 1969)

The previous chapter considered some of the challenges that health care professionals' face in providing palliative care that is appropriate, of high quality and yet remains meaningful to the dying person, their family and their carers. Professionals involved in such care are increasingly faced with ethical dilemmas as they seek to fulfil their respective caring goals. On the one hand quality is directly influenced by the changing circumstances of health care provision, which when combined with current advances and developments in health care treatments add increasing financial burden on currently limited budgets. On the other hand, subjective determinations of quality can be arrived at from the perspectives of the patients, their carers and their families. Those responsible for the provision of palliative care should be aware of the balance between perceived need and available resources, being equally responsible for managing budgets in a realistic manner and providing adequate resources to provide appropriate evidence-based standards of care. Within these parameters palliative care needs to be delivered professionally, within the law and be ethically permissible.

This chapter provides a discussion focusing on ethical issues at the end of life, in principle on the value and respect for life and how this influences decisions surrounding death and dying. Issues regarding honesty, truth-telling, coercion and collusion, while relevant at the end of life, are not expanded on. The chapter seeks to enable the reader to understand the basic building blocks behind ethical approaches to decision-making and through reflection to apply these to clinical situations toward the end of life.

In places suggestions are made for individual reflection on the issues surrounding the ethics involved. The reader is invited to reflect on these points and perhaps, where appropriate, to discuss them with a colleague or to read further about these points.

Since the first edition there have been developments impacting on ethical issues in palliative care. NICE (2004) guidance provided recommendations for the delivery of palliative care, with emphasis on promotion of the Gold Standards Framework (http://www.goldstandardsframework.nhs.uk/) (Thomas, 2003), focusing on organisation and delivery of palliative care services in the community; End of life Pathways (Ellershaw and Wilkinson, 2003), which further developed the concept of the Liverpool End of Life care Pathway (http://www.lcp-mariecurie.org.uk); and the Preferred Place of Care initiative (Lancashire and South Cumbria Cancer Services Network, 2003), promoting and enabling choice, which is now a key focus of client-orientated palliative care and governance. Legal regulations surrounding capacity, advanced decisions and lasting powers of attorney came into effect in April 2007 resulting from the Mental Capacity Act (2005), while legal issues about dying have been highlighted through the example of Diane Pretty, who requested that her partner be legally allowed to assist her to end her life (R (on the application of Pretty) v DPP). The challenge to ensure preference, choice and continuation of treatment was highlighted through Burke (Burke v UK (2006)), which indicted that in cases of treatment patients are unable to demand that specific interventions or treatments are continued. These, together with the debate surrounding the Assisted Dying for Terminally Ill People bill (House of Lords, 2005) have all been influential in the progression of palliative care services – and have the ability to further develop ethical issues in palliative care.

Initially this chapter will briefly consider the current influences on ethics in our society. This will inform the manner of the moral picture against which ethical decisions have to be made. Two key theories for determining whether the moral picture in our Western society is ethically permissible are outlined, these being *Consequentialism* and *Deontology*. Other theories could be considered, but for the sake of brevity and the more common approaches to health care, the justification of the moral argument has been restricted to these two. In determining the ethical permissibility of clinical situations the four key principles for health care ethics – respect for autonomy, beneficence, non-maleficence and justice – are introduced and examples used to illustrate the potential for conflict.

The temptation in determining what is ethically permissible is to consider the values held by the health care professionals in the situation, perhaps not deliberately ignoring the needs of the patient and their families, but not taking time to explore and consider the ethical implications of actions with them. Death is the one common denominator amongst all humans. Simone de Beauvoir (1969) recalled a comment made by her dying mother, quoted at the start of this chapter: 'Death does not frighten me; it is the jump I am afraid of'. The ethics involved perhaps need not focus on the morals of death but on the manner in which death is attained, the ethics behind the 'jump'.

Ethicists justify their decisions or argue their position and the validity of their reasoning by focusing on the overall moral picture and the ethical permissibility of their actions within the moral picture. Frequently the moral picture becomes complicated; the skill in ensuring that care is ethically permissible lies in determining what the actual moral picture being debated really is. Frequently conflict can arise in the ethical acceptability of the situation and subsequently in the desirability of some situations. One theoretical approach, Deontology, utilises a tool called the *Doctrine of Double Effect*, which permits Deontologists to find some actions ethically permissible despite certain foreseeable consequences that would not normally be justifiable for Deontologists. The *acts and omissions* doctrine suggests that under normal circumstances it is more ethically preferable to accept less favourable results of actions from omissions of care than to accept the same less favourable results from a deliberate action. There is contention (Rachels, 1975) that there remains no difference between actions or omissions of care, that there is no ethical difference in the intention to act or to omit care. This has particular relevance to the withholding and withdrawal of treatments, especially near the end of life. These latter two concepts will be outlined and applied to clinical examples to illustrate further potential for conflict and resolution within palliative health care provision.

Palliative care can lead perhaps to the greatest challenge, especially in determining ethical aspects of dying and of death. Health care professionals are aware of what they want to provide to maximise a person's quality of life, particularly where a person is dying. The focus of care is on improving the quality of life for the person and their family in the manner that is acceptable and wanted by the patient. Conflict might occur where the patient (perhaps in conjunction with their family) can feel that when they reach a point where their perception of their quality of life is so poor that in some circumstances death becomes a preferable option. Ending suffering is seen as more desirable than allowing the suffering to continue, despite whatever health care professionals may try to do to alleviate this. Randall and Downie (2006) challenge the purpose for tools used to determine and measure such a subjective quality – the quality of a person's life toward the end of their life – suggesting, perhaps slightly controversially, that such assessments should be abandoned as an aim of palliative care, with the focus being more on providing information to empower patients to participate in decisions, enable choice and hence reduce emotional distress. Such an approach supports the principles within health care ethics, but may be challenging in situations where the capacity of a person diminishes towards the end of their life.

The moral picture

This is the framework in which individuals or groups of people interact. Their actions or inactions have a direct effect on others, and result in the consequences of their actions or inactions. In ethics, the moral picture requires the individual to put aside emotive feelings about the subject and to engage in an objective discussion about the issues involved, depending on their particular philosophical school of thought. To illustrate the differences between Consequentialist and Deontological thinking, the following simplified moral picture should be considered.

A can do X to B with the result or outcome being Y

Consequentialist approaches

For Consequentialists, the prime consideration in determining whether something is ethically permissible or not is to look at the *consequences* in the moral picture. The ethical permissibility of the action (or inaction) X is determined on the acceptability of the consequences or outcome Y. For hedonistic Consequentialists acceptable consequences are those that maximise 'happiness' or benefit and minimise harm. There are other styles of Consequentialism or utilitarianism: *act-* and *rule-utilitarians*. Act-utilitarians consider the consequences for each individual moral picture, while rule-based utilitarians consider the moral picture, determine that which is ethically permissible and subsequently apply this to all similar situations.

Difficulties arise for Consequentialists in determining the overall benefit, as some actions can lead to both good and bad effects, and the benefit may be seen to be only from the perspective of those wishing the actions to be ethically permitted. Additional difficulty arises in determining the amount of benefit or minimum sadness. For example, if action X could distribute A to a greater number of B but with the outcome being that A is diluted and gives a limited 'happiness' to a great number, how might this compare with distributing A to a single recipient B where it could provide the maximum benefit, but only for that one person? Whose is the greater need? While both are good, is one of greater ethical permissibility? A final issue for Consequentialist determination depends on whether an individual or group decides that what gives them pleasure or happiness can only be obtained through X, which would be considered by others not to be a pleasure or happiness, or that their pleasure X is derived from a harm instigated on others.

The challenge for the Consequential approach to ethics is that some 'bad' actions may be considered ethically permissible if they lead to a perceived greater good in the outcome. It could be argued that a Consequentialist approach would argue that ending a life where there was tremendous suffering by active means could have a greater beneficial outcome for that individual. They would also argue that it could be equally permissible to end a life in order to save many others. Similarly, if there was a greater beneficial outcome a Consequentialist could argue that it would be ethically permissible to tell lies or steal if this would result in a greater beneficial outcome.

Deontological approaches

Deontologists, on the other hand, live according to categorical imperatives. Simply stated these are a set of rules or guidelines that govern their actions, for example not killing or not telling lies. The ethical permissibility of the moral picture focuses on the action X for which you are responsible. As long as X is ethically permissible then it is of no significance what the consequences or outcome Y become. The difficulty here is that adhering to some ethical principles as a deontologist can have disastrous consequences for others involved in the moral picture. A Deontological approach would find it ethically permissible not to end a life (not to kill) despite incredible suffering, even if there was a threat to end many lives. A Deontologist could not prevent that by killing the person who is about to carry out the threat. In Deontology ethically permitted situations would adhere in all circumstances to not killing, not telling lies, and not stealing. In these circumstances Deontology does not allow you to use a person as a means to an end. Where certain actions which are desirable in the moral picture might result in foreseeable consequences that are harmful, the Deontologist would refer to a tool known as the *Doctrine of Double Effect* (DDE) to determine whether the action was ethically permissible. This tool is often misquoted by the media; it could never make killing ethically acceptable for Deontologists.

Campbell and Collinson (1988, p. 153) offer an appropriate summary of the DDE:

> The Doctrine of Double Effect says that, on certain conditions, you need not be responsible for those effects of your actions which, though foreseen, are not intended.

In other words, it can make some actions ethically permissible that might have certain foreseeable side effects, provided that four conditions are met. These four conditions are (Campbell and Collinson, 1988, p. 155):

1. What is done must be, at the least, morally permissible.
2. What is intended must include only the good and not the bad effects of what is done.
3. The bad effects must not be the means whereby the good is brought about.
4. There must be proportionality between the good and the bad effects of what is done.

This becomes significant for Deontologists within palliative care, since this would ethically permit an action that would relieve suffering but which had a possible side effect of causing further harm to the patient.

Pause for thought I

■ How might a situation occur in palliative care where Deontologists use the DDE to ethically justify specific treatments, or the withdrawal of care?

The result of these two simplified outlines of Consequentialism and Deontology is that the differing approaches can both find ethically permissible actions or inactions that may be in conflict, particularly in the clinical situation. Health care professionals work within codes of conduct that govern their approaches to care. These generally require a duty of care to the patient. Subsequently health professionals' work can be greatly influenced from deontological perspectives. While the health care professional might perceive from the holistic nature of their palliative care that alternative consequences might be more desirable they can find that their care is governed and regulated by responsibilities and duties for which they become accountable.

An example of conflict that can arise between Deontologists and Consequentialists can be illustrated by the following.

A person enters an enclosed room where you are gathered with a large group of your colleagues and friends. She has a weapon, and she indicates that you have a choice: either you can end the lives of three members of the group, or she will end the lives of everyone in the room, leaving you until last.

Pause for thought 2

■ What would you do in such a situation?

■ Would your decisions change if the group of people changed (e.g. colleagues/strangers/close family/children/old people/patients/people who had been diagnosed with an incurable disease)?

■ How might your actions change and differ in your professional capacity? What influenced the change and why?

A consequential approach may be to recognise that, while the deaths of three members of the group is a harm, that this is offset by the saving of the lives of all the others in the group. The overall consequences are more beneficial than if everyone is killed; thus for a Consequentialist the decision to go along with the killing of three members of the group can be considered to be ethically permissible (to the relief of those who survive).

Should you hold stronger Deontological views, then you recognise that killing is not ethically permissible. Hence you are forced to choose the latter option offered by the terrorist. This results in the deaths of the entire group – but the decision that you made was ethically justifiable. The responsibility for the action of killing and for the deaths of the group remained with the person brandishing the gun.

This example illustrates how differing approaches to ethics can result in potential conflict, particularly where one approach finds that actions or inactions that can result in harm that is ethically permissible, while another approach could never consider such actions or inactions.

Principles of health care ethics

In determining whether the subject has received a benefit or a harm there are four key ethical principles that need to be considered. Identified by Beauchamp and Childress (1994) as the principles of *respect of autonomy*, *beneficence*, *non-maleficence* and *justice*, these principles form the ethical building blocks from which individual circumstances can be considered.

The principle of respect for autonomy

This is perhaps the strongest consideration in making clinical decisions. Respecting the autonomy of another requires that person to be actively involved in the decision-making process. Without such consultation, if the decisions are made on their behalf and for their benefit this may be considered paternalism. This is of particular relevance to dying people, because they can develop conditions or have decreased levels of consciousness in which they are unable to be consulted and to make informed knowledgeable decisions for themselves. In the absence of family members or friends who are then able to make decisions for that person, clinical decisions are left for the multi-professional team to determine. Their guide in making such decisions shall be to ensure that all decisions made for the patient are in the patient's best interests and that the patient would benefit from their decisions.

Gillon (1986, p. 60) defines autonomy as:

> ... the capacity to think, decide, and act on the basis of such thought and decision freely and independently and without ... let or hindrance.

Gillon further suggests that the key components to autonomy include the ability to think, the freedom of will to be able to do things that one wants, and finally to be able to perform one's desired wishes – the ability to act on those wishes.

Pause for thought 3

- How might the autonomy of a person who is dying be compromised?
- When might the paternalistic behaviour of health care professionals at the end of life be justified?
- How could the respect of the dying patient's autonomy be maximised in such circumstances?

Mind-altering chemicals can compromise autonomy, such as alcohol or certain medication. Autonomy may also be compromised by having the ability to choose one's circumstances removed or through coercion, or even the non-provision of sufficient information on which to make a choice.

As a person, you might have very strong preferences about how you might die and where. It is likely that you would consider these points to be very important, and while you are able to discuss and 'protect' your interests, your autonomy is likely to be respected. Unfortunately there are circumstances in which, through illness and disease, the person who is dying is less able to 'protect' their individual autonomy and as a result becomes increasingly vulnerable. This can be the result of either (a) the spread of the disease or illness and its effects on the manner in which the person is communicating their needs; (b) being physically unable to respond; or (c) being unable to understand the information and make decisions based upon the information. Autonomy is strongly related to consent, in that where autonomy is respected then health care professionals are required to obtain consent for the actions or procedures performed for a person.

The ability of people who are dying to maintain their autonomy can be diminished, particularly as they become increasingly unconscious. In the absence of a recent living will, families should be consulted as to what might be in the best interests of the patient; in the absence of close family or of a person appointed by the dying patient then health care professionals are forced to act in paternalistic manners. This encroaches on the autonomy of the patient while maintaining that no harm is done to the patient.

Beneficence and non-maleficence

At their simplest these principles are to do good and to do no harm respectively. There is some debate over which should take precedence. It would appear appropriate to do that which would cause no harm prior to that which obtains a good. It would be more appropriate to ensure that a dying person who was unable to communicate a preference had fewer harms inflicted on them rather than a momentary good.

Beneficence is, however, tempered by the principle of respect for autonomy of the patient, in that this is what the patient really wants. It is also tempered by non-maleficence – in that, in providing the benefit, would it cause a harm to be induced on others by depriving them of the opportunity? Finally, beneficence is tempered by the principle of justice; a harm may be perpetuated if the 'good' is not available for all. This respects the autonomy of others – health care professionals have autonomy and a right for their professional autonomy to be respected. They should not therefore be expected to perform actions that challenge the fairness of distribution.

Pause for thought 4

■ What makes a '*good*' good or preferable?
■ What makes a '*bad*' bad or harmful?
■ What influences our decisions in our everyday lives?
■ How might beneficence and non-maleficence influence factors at the end of life?

Non-maleficence in the care of the dying person can appear to be a desirable principle. However, there is a balance to the harms induced and their potential benefits. Individuals are normally happy to accept the sharp intra-muscular injections of analgesia for long-term pain relief. In palliative care, situations occur where what was considered ordinary treatment at an earlier stage in the patient's disease might be seen as extraordinary treatment near the end of life. The adverse side effects of chemotherapy are tolerated where there is hope of a beneficial cure for the disease. There are circumstances where in dying a person might elect to undergo a shorter-acting harm-inducing procedure where this is outweighed by the longer term benefit resulting from that procedure. Equally, the difficulty of ensuring beneficence or more of declining treatments to prevent further suffering could become of prime importance. This relates to the acts and omission doctrine, previously discussed, where Rachels argues that both have equal weighting in their moral outcome, and subsequently there is no moral difference between an action or an omission. It also relates to whether treatments can be considered to be ordinary or extraordinary in their means of treatment.

Justice

In ethics, justice is not the retributive style of justice but that of ensuring fairness and equality. This is difficult to maintain in a society and culture that are full of social inequalities. However, the principle remains that of equality for all, and what needs to be considered in coming to ethical decisions about actions or omissions is that, should an action or omission be provided for one person, then this should be available for all who wish to avail themselves of the action or omission of care. For those who are dying, this suggests that, whatever is done to care for one person should be provided for all other similar patients, and that there can be no place for the rationing of health care based on illness and disease, age or infirmity.

Pause for thought 5

- What are the resources that you control on a daily basis in your professional capacity?
- How do you decide how to distribute these resources?
- How do you ensure equality and equity in your distribution?

Paternalism

Paternalism is the making of decisions on the behalf of others in their best interests. Although intrinsically beneficial, paternalistic actions might not respect the individual autonomy of that person or group and may be seen not to respect their ability to choose for themselves given the appropriate information. A harmful action cannot be considered to be paternalistic, it remains a harm. Paternalism might not be considered to be ethically justifiable within a Deontological system. This could be considered to harm the rights of the person or group and therefore could not be considered to form the basis of a universal law. Consequentialists would consider the overall benefit to be derived from the situation and may find paternalistic action, in some instances, ethically permissible. However, in health care paternalism has been accepted where patients are unable to make decisions for themselves, particularly in situations where a person's 'competence' is diminished. This tends to reflect a consequential approach to decision making and can frequently occur within palliative care with the onset of unconsciousness, or of a person becoming increasingly unable to take decisions for themselves due to diseases affecting their ability to make rational decisions.

It could be argued that where a person's autonomy is diminished by circumstances that paternalism becomes increasingly justifiable, particularly where no other person has been appointed by the person to act a proxy consent. At times, though, decisions are made on the patient's behalf citing that the person could not understand the information required. The issue here is whether the person has actually been consulted, offered the choice of whether they wish to know, or even if the information can be simplified while retaining accuracy in order for them to understand it better and come to their own decision. Time is a large factor in such situations, but needs to be made available, particularly within palliative care.

Pause for thought 6

- Could paternalism be used to justify withdrawal of care in the end of life situations?
- What steps could be taken to try to minimise paternalistic actions at the end of life?
- To what extent are you aware of paternalistic action being adopted within your area of work (does this extend to meal times, taking vital signs etc?)

Clinical decisions

As with all aspects of health care, perhaps of paramount ethical importance in palliative care is to respect the autonomy of the individual. This can be achieved by at least attempting to maximise the opportunity for the patient to receive information, to understand, to come to a personal decision and to communicate their decision freely. Many situations in clinical conditions can involve difficulties in ensuring that this is always possible. Difficulties may result from either the competence of the patient being diminished or through the paternalistic behaviour of health care providers. Even where the patient is competent and fulfils the abilities described above, he or she can come to a decision that he/she may consider the quality of his/her life to be minimal, and that his/her personal condition maximises suffering. In such instances it can be understandable why an individual might choose a decision that he would prefer his life to end. This is a very individual decision, best made in consultation with close family in order that they can understand the patient's reasoning, and is by no means an easy one to come to (or so I would imagine). Ultimately this must represent a failure of care – physical, psychological, emotional, social and spiritual – to maximise the quality of life for the patient, to enable them to live until they die. Such decisions challenge the ethics of health care in that carers are unable to provide what the patient requires. Health care professionals could not act on a declaration of wanting life to end, even when made by a fully autonomous person. They are bound by their professional codes of conduct not to harm (e.g. by the ending of a life) patients. This may not be as clear cut for health care professionals as they might like, particularly where they hold personal Consequentialist views. A carer may see as harmful the continued and prolonged suffering endured by the dying patient and family in situations where adequate palliative care is not provided or sufficient to maintain the quality of life for the patient who is dying.

It could be considered that in some instances the health service is keeping people alive beyond points where their physical bodies can hope to repair. There is a recognisable difference between stopping the working of a ventilator following the criteria for brain stem death being satisfied and the situation of a person who has a diagnosis of being in a persistent vegetative state, when the equivalent ending of life (even with the agreement of family) by withholding food could be considered a harm. The withholding of food would be an omission of care; a withdrawal of the means by which the patient was fed would be an action (e.g. removal of a feeding tube). It ensures a slower death by the removal of that which was maintaining the patient. Is there a moral difference between the action of switching off a ventilator and the removal of a feeding tube? In one case parts of the brain are able to function unaided, while in the other the parts of the brain essential to maintain life are irrecoverably damaged. There is a difference in comparing the category of patient. It would appear that where the body's vital signs are naturally maintained then this is taken as being of sufficient interest to warrant closer attention and consideration of whether that life can be ethically ended by deliberate action. The situation needs to determine whether the care of the dying person is by ordinary or extraordinary means, and where the boundary crosses from being ordinary to extraordinary treatments for dying people.

Pause for thought 7

- What constitutes ordinary care and extraordinary care for a person who is dying?
- Who is likely to determine this?
- When and how might ordinary care become extraordinary care at the end of life?
- What determines how far extraordinary care is offered to dying people?
- How might this influence the quality of their life, and of their dying?
- If the extraordinary care cannot be offered to every person who wants it, should it be offered at all?

Death and dying

In considering the ethics surrounding dying and death the question of whether a difference exists between the two states needs to be addressed. Should greater value be placed on life? Death is the unknown factor, an event of which the majority of people are aware.

> Human death is an unknown, surrounded by myth, dreams, fears, uncertainties and distress of all kinds (Campbell *et al.*, 1997)

Death is a distinct event that every human will encounter, a certainty that might not respect individual autonomous wishes. Can death have ethical considerations? If value is placed on living then there should be equal value on the manner of dying or on the ending of life. If life should be respected, then it would be appropriate to respect the manner of dying. While death is a certainty, there is no choice about it. It is the vulnerability of individuals who are dying that needs to be recognised. It is for this reason that health care workers should consider the ethical basis of their care and of how decisions about that care are arrived at in order not to take advantage of the vulnerable person.

Death can be both beneficial and non-maleficent, particularly where it offers a release from suffering. Above all it is perhaps the most accurate and appropriately distributed notion of justice that could be considered: it comes to everyone.

Perhaps it is not death that has strong ethical connections but the manner in which death arrives that has the greater ethical significance. Neuberger (1999) places emphasis on recognising the spiritual aspects of dying within care provided. She encourages a societal change to the subject of death and dying to make the face of death more acceptable and less frightening:

> We will only achieve a real change, allowing ourselves to express our fears and hopes and desires if we are able and prepared to face the issue of how best to meet our end, and the end of others we love and respect, by discussing, talking, arguing, planning, and by resolving to improve what is still a very patchy situation in this country, where we only get the chance of having a good death by battling against the odds.

Death can be the result of natural old age, disease, natural accidents and disasters. In the latter cases we consider these deaths 'acts of God' and are perhaps relieved that we were not in that part of creation to experience the phenomenon, but are duly reminded of our frail mortality. Death that arrive through accidents and unforeseeable consequences are seen as being unfortunate and untimely. Under these circumstances death is neutral, the ending of life through natural and unplanned action. Death can also be brought about by deliberate circumstance: killing through war, suicide, sacrifice, murder and euthanasia and by capital punishment. Is there a difference between the ethical notions of the manner in which death is brought about?

This issue could be considered as to what is morally wrong with death. Glover (1977) would suggest that there is little wrong with death, only in killing. Killing does not become a wrong in that it deprives a person of his/her intrinsic value of his/her life, but that killing is wrong in that it reduces the length of a 'worthwhile' life. Killing of a person who would want to go on living is wrong, or to kill in a manner that causes fear or harm prior to the death. Killing is also wrong due to the harmful effect on those left behind and the deprivation of the dead person's contribution to society (among other things). In the same way that killing can be seen to be a moral bad, the saving of life then becomes increasingly morally acceptable; thus it becomes harder to ethically justify the hastening of death whatever the circumstances.

Pause for thought 8

- What makes life and living 'worthwhile'?
- How might you determine at what point a life is considered to not be 'worthwhile' at the end of life?

However, the notion of killing has differing degrees of acceptability. The killing of another child or elderly person unable to defend themselves is considered perhaps worse than that of a person who could defend themselves. The killing of self, until 1961, was considered by law to be an illegal act. In contrast, self-killing could be considered to be more valuable in the sacrificial sense where the lives of others are saved – for example, the fighter pilot who does not eject from a stricken plane in order to ensure that it does not crash into a village, a case of a person who saves the life of another but in doing so recognises that he is putting his own life at great risk. The manner of these deaths appears to be ethically preferable to others, in that the death gains value. There remains the ethical question of whether the manner of this death is ethically acceptable, or as ethically acceptable as suicide. If this is more ethically acceptable, then how should the views of a mother or father wishing to donate their heart (given it to be a perfect match) for their only child be considered?

The difference between these manners of killing becomes one of how benefit is measured, and whether there is proportionality between the two sets of circumstances. The consequences become valuable in determining the ethical permissibility. While accepted by Consequentialists, Deontologists use the DDE to find such actions ethically permissible. What tends to determine whether the manner of death is morally acceptable in the eyes of society can too often be the resultant of misplaced media misinformation. The manner of dying, however, can appear to be on the surface more acceptable in some guises.

The taking of a life is morally wrong. It deprives the person of his/her life, it deprives others of the person's continued contribution to their lives and it does not respect the autonomy of the person if they do not wish to die at that moment.

There are circumstances in which a patient chooses to die, to retain their right to choose to end their life. Where competent, this is an autonomous choice and can be respected as a decision. The NCHSPCS (1997) recognised the right of the individual to wish to die; however the challenge for health care professionals occurs where the wish becomes a request to assist in the hastening of death for a patient. This situation remains illegal within English law. It crosses the divide of what is ethically permissible, particularly for Deontologists. While we need to respect the autonomy of others, which can include their wish to die, this has to be tempered with their respect of our own autonomy in not wishing to kill a person.

While the moral wrongness of *killing* is recognised by Glover (1977), who offers a sound argument as to why it is ethically wrong to take a life, another ethical consideration is what *value* life has. If life has value then it becomes unethical to deprive a person of it. Harris (1985) considers that which makes life valuable is not based on equity across all people but the capacity to value the lives of ourselves and of others. Subsequently the inherent wrong of killing is to deprive a person of the capacity to value their lives. While this argument supports the notion that the ending of a life is wrong in itself, there is another consideration for this point. Where a person does not value his life, can depriving him of life be considered to be morally wrong? It is then perhaps that it is the manner of dying that becomes important. The issue of Harris's capacity for life also becomes important in consideration of dying: does a person have capacity to appreciate the manner in which they are dying, and if they do not have that capacity then would it be ethically acceptable to deprive them of their life by killing them?

While capacity to value is appropriate for those who are competent to determine and articulate what they want, there is an issue for those whose personal autonomy is restricted, for example unconscious people. The Mental Capacity Act (2005) recognises the status of advanced decisions (which have been previously recognised as living wills) to enable the wishes of the person to be stated at the point in time that the living will is written. While not indicating current wishes, the advance directive will indicate preference for choice of treatment or refusal of treatments and will provide insight into the feelings and wishes of patients. Advanced decisions can indicate the preferences of the dying person, and combined with lasting power of attorney relating to welfare of the individual, could enable a client to maintain some control over their care should they not be able to communicate their wishes toward the end of their life. Advanced decisions will not be able to include directions to actually end the life of the person; this could not be ethically (or legally) permitted and should be ignored by carers. Advanced decisions will offer insight into a person's preferences and an indication of what the person does or does not want; unlike living wills they have recognition within the Act and subsequently are set to become increasingly legally binding. The implications for practice are that professionals will need to determine at an early stage whether an individual has a current advanced decision, and whether a client has appointed someone with their lasting power of attorney.

The ethical discussions surrounding euthanasia, or more appropriately active suicide, have recently been a focus for contemporary palliative care ethics. Lord Joffe's Assisted Dying for the Terminally Ill Bill (HL 2005) recognised the real challenges and choices faced by some individuals towards the end of their lives and promoted discussion about safeguards for vulnerable groups, the impact on relationships between professionals, carers and patients, and the potential impact on palliative care services should assisted dying become legalised (NCPC, 2006). At the end of the debate the situation remains that assisted dying remains unlawful. While many argue that this is ethically acceptable we have to recognise that for some individuals this leaves them with a choice of having to travel to places where assisted voluntary euthanasia is legalised, which necessitates a journey while they are still physically able to do so, perhaps depriving a person of additional 'quality' time at the end of their lives in their own homes if that was their preferred choice.

The ethical permissibility in this area focuses on the quality of life versus the sanctity of life. Currently in English law there is a prohibition on the killing or deliberate taking of a human life. The professional bodies for health care professionals reflect this Deontological sentiment, placing emphasis on a duty of care, and of not harming a patient. This works for Deontological style ethicists, but for those of consequential persuasion there is a balance between the quality of life (that which makes a life worthwhile) and its duration and extent of imposed 'suffering' compared with the implication of hastening the end of that life. Both notions require an ethical justification of the value of life based on ethical principles.

The ethics surrounding palliative care is frequently dominated by the debate surrounding euthanasia, which is a worthwhile debate in itself. The arguments against allowing assisted dying or assisted voluntary euthanasia are adequately summarised by Finlay *et al.* (2005), who focus on the sanctity of life, the value of life and the implications for palliative care services should such a law come into effect.

By its definition, palliative care neither hastens nor prolongs death (Twycross, 1999). Successive definitions of palliative care have all focused on the nature of palliative care being active and holistic, delivered by a multi-professional team and focused on patients and their families experiencing an advanced progressive illness. The recognition of the goal of palliative care being related to the 'best quality of life' was recognised by WHO (2002), but Randall and Downie (2006) would suggest that this is too subjective and difficult to quantify within palliative care – rather than determining whether palliative care ethics focus on quality issues they suggest that the focus ought to be on providing opportunities that support and empower choice.

The National Council for Palliative Care indicate the aims of palliative care to include 'affirm living and dying as a normal process' (NCPC, 2006). Euthanasia suggests the ending of life by passive or active means, in the voluntary or non-voluntary capacities of the dying person. It suggests a premature ending of life which is in conflict with the ethos of palliative care. Subsequently in palliative care there can be little consideration for active voluntary euthanasia apart from recognising the potential influences that it exerts on the provision of high-quality care. The only debatable potential for consideration within palliative care could be where caring professionals respect the autonomous wishes of a dying person not to commence further treatments but to continue to provide the basic care required. This omission of 'care' is perhaps as close to passive, voluntary euthanasia that palliative care could ever get to.

Concluding thoughts

The sanctity of life would appear to mirror the value of life, and where the value of life is it should not be prematurely ended. The ethics of dying and death need to consider the individual manner of dying and the person's fears, concerns and other wishes. It would be ethically more preferable to work to maintain the dying person's quality of life, while recognising the individual nature of death and the circumstances surrounding dying and death. Careful consideration of the ethics involved in differing situations enable ethically based permissible care to be provided. Dame Cicely Saunders commented on the importance of caring for those who are dying, recognising that what becomes important is enabling someone to live until they die. Appropriate consideration of ethical principles, together with recognition of how they are being applied, can enable carers to provide ethically justifiable actions or omissions that enable patients to live their lives more fully to the point where they die.

Randall and Downie (1999, p. 304) in discussion about the value of life conclude that 'Values are in the end personal preferences, but ethics is a system of interpersonal rules for the better ordering of human life'. In determining the ethics of dying well, careful consideration of ethical rules, recognition of where they have come from and their influences on our personal lives should ensure that the care offered to those who are dying and their families is not just justifiable and permissible, but appropriate for that person while remaining within professional boundaries.

The principles of health care ethics provide the building blocks on which the moral picture can be explored, while ethical theory provides the framework in determining the acceptability (or not) of decisions and care, be it action or omission. Carers need to utilise ethics to protect the vulnerable dying person, and to maximise the benefits in maintaining the person's quality of life.

References

Beauchamp, T. L. and Childress, J. F. (1994) *Principles of Biomedical Ethics*, 4th edn. Oxford University Press, Oxford.

Campbell, A., Charlesworth, M., Gillett, G. and Jones, G. (1997) *Medical Ethics*, 2nd edn. Oxford University Press, Oxford.

Campbell, R. and Collinson, D. (1988) *Ending Lives*. Blackwell, Oxford.

De Beauvoir, S. (1969) *A Very Easy Death*. Penguin, London.

Ellershaw, J. and Wilkinson, S. (eds) (2003) *Care of the Dying: a Pathway to Excellence*. Oxford University Press, Oxford.

Finlay, I. G., Wheatley, V. J. and Izdebski, C. (2005) The House of Lords Select Committee on the Assisted Dying for the Terminally Ill Bill: implications for specialist palliative care. *Palliative Medicine*, **19**, 444–53.

Gold Standards Framework (unknown) *The Gold Standards Framework; a Programme for Community Palliative Care*. Available online from http://www.goldstandardsframework.nhs.uk (Accessed 28 November 2006).

Gillon, R. (1986) *Philosophical Medical Ethics*. John Wiley & Sons, Chichester.

Glover, J. (1977) *Causing Death and Saving Lives*. Penguin, London.

Harris, J. (1985) *The Value of Life: an Introduction to Medical Ethics*. Routledge, London.

House of Lords Select Committee (2005) *The Assisted Dying for the Terminally Ill Bill. HL. London The Stationery Office*. Available online from http://www.publications.parliament.uk/pa/ld200506/ldbills/036/2006036.htm (Accessed 28 November 2006).

Lancashire and South Cumbria Cancer Services Network (2003) *The Preferred Place of Care Plan*. Available online from http://www.cancerlancashire.org.uk/ppc.html (Accessed 28 November 2006).

Liverpool Care Pathway (2003) *The Liverpool Care Pathway for the Dying Patient (LCP)*. Available online from http://www.lcp-mariecurie.org.uk/about/ (Accessed 28 November 2006).

The Mental Capacity Act (2005) HMSO, London.

NCHSPCS (1997) *Voluntary Euthanasia: The Council's View*. NCHSPCS, London.

National Council for Palliative Care (unknown) *Palliative Care Explained.* Available online from http://www.ncpc.org.uk/palliative_care.html (Accessed 28 November 2006).

NCPC (2006) *Response to: The Assisted Dying for the Terminally Ill Bill 2005.* NCPC, London.

NICE (2004) *Guidance on Cancer Services. Improving Supportive and Palliative Care for Adults with Cancer.* NICE, London.

Neuberger, J. (1999) *Dying Well: a Guide to Enabling A Good Death.* Hochland and Hochland, Hale.

Randall, F. and Downie, R. (1999) *Palliative Care Ethics: a Companion for All Specialities,* 2nd edn. Oxford University Press, Oxford.

Randall, F. and Downie, R. (2006) *The Philosophy of Palliative Care: Critique and Reconstruction.* Oxford University Press, Oxford.

Rachels, J. (1975) Active and passive euthanasia. New England Journal of Medicine, **292**, 78–80, cited by Gillon, R. (1986) *Philosophical Medical Ethics.* John Wiley and Sons, Chichester.

Thomas, K. (2003) *Caring from the Dying at Home: Companions on the Journey.* Radcliffe Medical Press, Abingdon.

Twycross, R. (1999) *Introducing Palliative Care,* 3rd edn. Radcliffe Medical Press, Abingdon.

World Health Organization (2002) *National Cancer Control Programmes: Policies and Guidelines.* WHO, Geneva.

Legal cases

R (on the application of Pretty) v DPP [2002] 1 All ER 1

R (Burke) v GMC [2005] EWCA 1003 and Burke v UK (2006)

CHAPTER 7

Dying by euthanasia: an easy thing to do?

Hilde de Vocht

Introduction

As a Dutch researcher in palliative care I regularly attend conferences abroad. No matter what the topic of my presentation is, delegates invariably tend to ask me about euthanasia. Such questions and subsequent discussion make one realise how the Netherlands has become the focus of attention when it comes to euthanasia. Admittedly, the Netherlands was the first country in the world to legalise euthanasia and assisted suicide. Sadly though, I sometimes find that people are not very well informed on Dutch legislation and its practice with regard to euthanasia and assisted suicide. The media, which have a wider reach and influence, do not always inform their public accurately on the position of euthanasia in the Netherlands. A possible explanation for this may be that the sources for their information are not credible, and therefore do not reflect the reality of the Dutch euthanasia situation. Another explanation, although extreme, may be that the media deliberately misrepresent the euthanasia position in the Netherlands as a way of discouraging other countries from legalising the practice. I believe the media and other sources have a duty to provide the public with accurate information. I am therefore grateful to have this opportunity to write this chapter as a platform to present more accurate information on euthanasia and assisted suicide in the Netherlands. It can be argued that this information can then be used as a basis for formulating individual opinions and choices about end of life decisions. Worldwide, more and more countries are challenged to discuss the topic, with a view to legalising euthanasia and assisted suicide. The recent debate on the amended version of Lord Joffe's Assisted Dying Bill (2006) in the House of Lords in the UK serves as a good example.

This chapter begins by offering the reader comprehensive information on Dutch legislation and practice with regard to euthanasia and assisted suicide. Much of this information can also be found in English on the site of the Right to Die-NL (http://www.nvve.nl/) and the site of the euthanasia review committees (http://www.toetsingscommissieseuthanasie.nl/). Attention is paid to the national and international debate and to the ethical perspective. Finally, the question of whether or not dying by euthanasia is an easy thing to do will be addressed.

Definition of euthanasia and assisted suicide: what it is and what it is not

In the Netherlands, euthanasia has officially been defined as: 'intentionally terminating another person's life at that person's request' (Staatscommissie, 1985, p. 26). Assisted suicide is defined as 'helping another person to terminate his or her life'. In Dutch law these two terms are generally treated together. There are clear guidelines and criteria to be satisfied before carrying out euthanasia or assisted suicide. The same statutory criteria of due care and the same notification procedure are required for euthanasia and assisted suicide if physicians want to make sure they will not be prosecuted. Having said this, the main focus of this chapter will be on euthanasia.

Now that the definitions are clear it also becomes logical that euthanasia and assisted suicide should be distinguished from other end-of-life decisions (Besse *et al.*, 2006), which, in the Netherlands, are part of normal medical practice, such as:

- Refusal of treatment: a patient who is mentally competent may refuse his or her consent for the start or continuation of medical treatment. The physician in question must respect that decision, even if it results in or speeds up the patient's death.
- Withholding or withdrawing medically futile treatment: this requires a medical opinion on whether further treatment has any point. In such situations, the physician should consult with colleagues to ensure that the decision is as objective as possible.
- Adequate pain control: a physician may attempt to relieve pain using stronger medication, even if this may have the side effect of hastening death. Dosages should be in accordance with the goal of pain control.
- Palliative sedation: this is the deliberate lowering of a patient's level of consciousness in the last stages of life. There are no indications that palliative sedation will hasten death. The patient will die from the progress of the disease he is suffering from.

In cases of deep sedation that is meant to be continued until the patient dies, fluids and food are often withheld, as it would serve no medical purpose to administer them. According to the official Dutch guidelines for palliative sedation, this is acceptable if the patient is not expected to survive longer than one to two weeks (KNMG, 2005).

Euthanasia has one goal: the dignified death of the patient at his request. All the other above-mentioned decisions are about not prolonging life, which is different from terminating life. The difference is that, if life is not prolonged, patients die as a result of their illness. When life is terminated, people die as a result of an active intervention.

As a consequence of this there is no such thing as 'passive euthanasia' in the Netherlands and the use of this expression gives rise to a lot of confusion. Anything that is called 'passive euthanasia' does not involve actively terminating someone's life and therefore does not fit the Dutch definition of euthanasia. There is, by definition, only one form of euthanasia, that is, the 'active' form of euthanasia, and therefore no need to use the adjective 'passive' in this context.

The Termination of Life on Request and Assisted Suicide Act

On 10 April 2001, the Dutch parliament passed a new Act on euthanasia: the Termination of Life on Request and Assisted Suicide (Review Procedures) Act (http://www.nvve.nl/assets/nvve/english/euthlawenglish.pdf). It came into effect on 1 April 2002. This did not change the original position that euthanasia and assisting a person in committing suicide are criminal offences with maximum terms of imprisonment of twelve and three years respectively. Since the new Act was passed, however, the relevant articles of the Dutch Criminal Code contain special grounds for immunity from criminal liability, and these apply only to physicians. Physicians who comply with a request for euthanasia or assisted suicide are exempt from prosecution provided they fulfil the statutory criteria of due care and notify the authorities in the prescribed manner. These due care criteria and the required notification procedure are described in the next paragraphs.

Statutory criteria of due care

An independent review committee assesses whether a physician has met the due care criteria. A thorough comprehension of these criteria is a prerequisite to understanding which standards a review committee uses to arrive at its conclusion. Box 7.1 contains an outline of what constitutes due care and must be adhered to by all participating physicians.

Box 7.1 Statutory criteria of due care

A physician who ends a patient's life must:

- be convinced that the patient's request is voluntary, well-considered and lasting;
- be convinced that the patient's suffering is unbearable and that there is no prospect of improvement;
- inform the patient of his or her situation and prospects;
- discuss the situation with the patient and come to the joint conclusion that there is no reasonable alternative;
- consult at least one other physician with no connection to the case;
- carry out the procedure in a medically appropriate fashion.

Source: http://www.nvve.nl/assets/nvve/english/euthlawenglish.pdf

Statutory criteria of due care elaborated

A physician who ends a patient's life must:

- *Be convinced that the patient's request is voluntary, well-considered and lasting*
  The basic precondition for justifiable termination of life or assisted suicide is the patient's explicit request. It is not permitted to comply with a request that has been made on impulse in a highly emotional state. For a request to be voluntary, no pressure or influence must be exerted on the patient. Although family and often nursing staff and caregivers are involved in the request, they do not have to agree with it. The patient's wishes are paramount. A request is well considered if the patient has a full understanding of his illness. This includes understanding of the diagnosis, prognosis and treatment options.

  Only patients capable of expressing their wishes may request euthanasia or assistance with suicide and they must do so in person. This rules out requests from parents or a legal representative. Under the Act, minors aged

12 or over may however make such a request. In line with existing rules on medical procedures relating to minors, the Act distinguishes between two age categories. Patients between the ages of 12 and 16 need the consent of their parents or guardian. Sixteen and 17-year-olds can in principle make an independent request, although their parents or guardian must be involved in the decision-making process.

■ *Be convinced that the patient's suffering is unbearable and that there is no prospect of improvement*
The absence of prospects for improvement must be determined according to prevailing medical opinion. Physicians claim that, in the medical sense, this can be established fairly objectively. The physician's professional opinion on the scope for treatment and care plays a major role.

It is more difficult to establish whether suffering is unbearable, because this is person-related (subjective). It is determined by the patient's outlook on life, meaning, their physical and mental strength and their personality. What one person regards as bearable may be unbearable for another. Readers interested in the notion of suffering are referred to Cassell (1992) and Nyatanga (2005) for a detailed discussion. However, for a third person to assess whether suffering is unbearable, there has to be some kind of objective standard. The committee therefore examines whether the physician found the patient's suffering palpably unbearable. The committee bases its judgement on the report the physician has to write and in which he justifies how due care was exercised (see 'Notification procedure and follow up').

■ *Inform the patient of his or her situation and prospects*
In assessing this due care criterion, the committee examines whether and how the physician informed the patient of his illness and prognosis. For patients to make a well-considered request, they need to have a full understanding of their illness, the diagnosis, prognosis and possible treatment. It is the physician's responsibility to ensure that the patient is fully informed, and to verify that. Meeting this criterion is a prerequisite for meeting the next criterion.

■ *Discuss the situation with the patient and come to a joint conclusion that there is no reasonable alternative*
The physician and the patient must be convinced that there is no alternative other than euthanasia or assisted suicide. This criterion makes it clear that the decision-making process is a matter involving both patient and physician.

The main priority is the care and treatment of the patient, and for his suffering to be discussed and relieved as far as possible. The question is whether there are prospects for improving the patient's situation within a reasonable time and whether the results of treatment warrant the 'burden' and side effects endured by the patient.

The provision of good medical treatment (including palliative care) is the essence of the physician–patient relationship. Euthanasia is the final resort and only becomes an issue once the patient and physician are convinced that there are no longer any realistic prospects for treatment. That does not mean to say that every possible type of palliative treatment must be tried first. Some forms of treatment have side effects that are difficult for patients to tolerate. Radiotherapy can have such serious side effects, like vomiting and alopecia, that the disadvantages of treatment outweigh the advantages. Some patients refuse further palliative treatment – in the form, for instance, of palliative sedation – because they absolutely do not want to become drowsy or lose consciousness. For example, those with a strong Buddhist persuasion believe that it is paramount to have clear consciousness till death (Nyatanga, 2001).

There may therefore be good reasons to refrain from further treatment. If treatment is refused, the committee decides on a case-by-case basis whether there was 'no reasonable alternative'. Because physician and patient come to a joint decision, physicians are expected to indicate in their report why the patient's refusal of an alternative treatment was reasonable in that situation and at that time.

- *Consult at least one other physician with no connection to the case, who must then meet the patient and state in writing that the attending physician has satisfied the due care criteria listed in the four points above*
  The consultation criterion requires that the physician consults at least one other physician who has no connection either with him or the patient. This physician must have seen the patient and given a written opinion on whether the due care criteria have been observed.

  It is emphasised that this physician must be an independent colleague, neither a member of the same practice or partnership, nor a relative, intern or any other physician in a subordinate position to the attending physician. The consulting physician must familiarise himself with the patient's medical situation and his request by visiting the patient and if necessary examining him.

  The independent physician's report, containing a description of the patient's condition at the time of the visit and of his/her wishes as expressed at that time, is essential to the committee's assessment. He must also state how he determined whether all the due criteria had been fulfilled, and give reasons for his conclusions. He should also describe explicitly the (absence of) a relationship with the patient and the attending physician. The Royal Netherlands Medical Association (KNMG) offers special training for physicians to provide a second opinion in cases of requests for euthanasia.

- *Carry out the procedure in a medically appropriate fashion*
  The preferred method to carry out euthanasia is by using intravenous infusion (Besse *et al.*, 2006). An anaestheticum (thiopental natrium) is administered to induce a coma and a muscle relaxant (pancuronium or vecuronium)

makes respirations cease and stops the heart from beating. An alternative method is to give the patient two injections, the first one with thiopental natrium and the second one with pancuronium or vecuronium.

In assisted suicide the physician usually gives the patient a liquid consisting of a barbiturate overdose in combination with sugar and alcohol. After drinking the liquid the patient falls asleep and dies as a result of respiration seizure and the heart stopping beating. The physician must be present when the patient drinks the liquid and must stay with him/her until death occurs. Leaving the drugs for self-administration without supervision is risky and medically irresponsible.

The criterion that due medical care and attention must be exercised has two components:
- The right drugs must be administered in the correct manner.
- They must be administered by the attending physician himself and not left to nursing staff.

Notification procedure and follow-up

After the death of the patient, the physician who carried out euthanasia must immediately notify the municipal pathologist of this instance of death from non-natural causes. The pathologist then performs a post mortem examination to determine how euthanasia was performed and what means were used. He compiles a report on his findings. This report is sent to the public prosecutor. If there are no irregularities, the public prosecutor will give permission for the body to be released for burial or cremation.

The physician himself has to write a report in which he justifies how due care was exercised in this specific case of euthanasia or assisted suicide.

The pathologist's report and the physician's report are submitted to the regional review committee. There are five such committees in the Netherlands. Each review committee has an odd number of members and includes a legal expert (who acts as chair), a physician and an expert on ethical issues. The committee assesses whether the physician met the statutory due care criteria. If it finds that he failed to do so, or may have failed to do so, it notifies the Board of Procurators of the Public Prosecution Service and the regional health care inspector of its findings. These bodies then decide on the basis of their own competence and responsibility whether further legal or disciplinary steps need to be taken.

Starting in May 2006, all the cases that are reviewed by the review committees have their findings published through a data bank on the Internet that can be accessed by anyone. All details of the cases can be found here, while ensuring anonymity of patients. One of the aims of publishing the committees' findings is to improve physicians' understanding of the working methods of the committees and thereby to increase their willingness to report cases. It is hoped that publishing these findings will also further improve the quality of procedures for the termination of life. Another purpose is to demonstrate that physicians in the Netherlands handle euthanasia and assisted suicide with great care and great concern for the uniqueness and individuality of each death. Unfortunately, for non-Dutch speaking readers, this data bank is only available in Dutch. A few cases (in English) from the Annual Report 2005 (Regionale toetsingscommissies euthanasie, 2006) have been included in this chapter.

What numbers are we talking about?

In the Netherlands, about 10,000 requests for euthanasia are made each year (see http://www.nvve.nl/). Not every request eventually leads to euthanasia. Two-thirds of the requests for euthanasia made to physicians are refused for different reasons. For example, there may still be treatment options that offer some hope of improving the patient's condition. There may be ways of relieving a patient's suffering, such as more effective pain control, to be tried first before granting the euthanasia request. Many patients die before a decision is reached on their request for euthanasia. Sometimes, patients find sufficient peace of mind in the knowledge that the physician is prepared to perform euthanasia if necessary and may never go ahead with their requests.

In 2005 a total 136,402 people died in the Netherlands (http://www.cbs.nl/). This figure includes 1933 deaths notified to the euthanasia review committees. Out of the 1933 deaths, there were 1765 cases of euthanasia, 143 cases of assisted suicide and 25 cases involving a combination of the two. From these figures, it can be seen that the percentage of reported euthanasia was 1.3% of the total deaths in the Netherlands. The percentage for all reported cases of euthanasia and/or assisted suicide was 1.4%. The point to make here is that, while euthanasia is permissible in the Netherlands, there is only a small percentage of deaths by euthanasia/assisted suicide when compared to the total number of deaths per year. Moreover, the frequency of euthanasia and assisted suicide has decreased considerably over the last few years; there does not seem to be any question of a slippery slope with regard to life termination (ZonMw, 2007).

Just to give an idea: the percentage of suicides (unassisted) during 2005 in the Netherlands was 1.2%. There are a greater number of people who died an unnatural death with medical assistance than people committing suicide without such help.

Table 7.1 shows an overview of the disease/disorders for the 1933 patients who died of euthanasia and or assisted suicide in 2005. Table 7.2 shows the location of euthanasia carried out in 2005.

Table 7.1 Overview of patient disease/disorders in 2005 (Regionale toetsingscommissies euthanasie, 2006).

Cancer	1713
Cardiovascular disease	23
Neurological disorders	85
Pulmonary disorders, other than cancer	29
Other (including AIDS)	27
Combination of diseases	56

Table 7.2 Location of euthanasia/assisted suicide in 2005 (Regionale toetsingscommissies euthanasie, 2006).

At own home	1585
Hospital	159
Nursing home	73
Care home	44
Another institution	6
Elsewhere (e.g. in a hospice or at the home of a relative)	66

The review committees reviewed all 1933 cases. In three cases the committees found that the attending physician had not acted in accordance with the due care criteria while carrying out euthanasia. In these three cases the matter was referred to the Board of Procurators General and the Health Care Inspectorate.

Below, two cases of euthanasia are presented showing how due care criteria were adhered to and also what happens when they are not followed. The cases also show how the attending physician assesses, consults others and later reports to the review committee after carrying out euthanasia.

Cases of euthanasia: two examples

Case 1

Case 1 illustrates how notifications are assessed by the review committee for fulfilment of the due care criteria. This case is an existing case that can be found in the Annual Report of the Euthanasia Review Committees 2005. In practically every case, including this one, the committees found that the physician acted in accordance with the due care criteria.

In June 2005 the patient, a 58-year-old woman, was diagnosed with occlusive icterus due to a tumour in the head of the pancreas. Before a final diagnosis could be made she suffered a perforated intestine and peritonitis, for which she underwent surgery involving the insertion of a stent. The patient suffered severe post-operative complications. There was no prospect of recovery. Scans revealed that the tumour was getting larger and that the patient had pulmonary metastases. She was given maximum pain relief (300 micrograms of Durogesic a day, and extra morphine by nasal tube if necessary).

The patient was suffering from increasing pain despite efforts to relieve it, increasing nausea, ascites and the fact that she could only be fed by nasal tube. She found this suffering unbearable.

Apart from the palliative measures already in place, there were no other ways to alleviate her suffering. The documents indicate that the physician gave her sufficient information about her situation and prognosis. He expected her to die soon.

The patient made her first specific request for euthanasia in September 2005, and repeated this request several times thereafter.

The physician called in an independent general practitioner who was trained to give a second opinion in case of a request for euthanasia. After obtaining information about the patient from the notifying physician, the independent physician saw her for the first time in late September 2005 and again a month later. In his report he described the patient's case history and confirmed that the specialists treating her had said she would not survive major surgery. His report stated that she was extremely debilitated, somewhat cachectic and bedridden. She could only just manage to go to the toilet unaided. The patient said she was anxious to get her affairs properly organised, as she wanted to avoid a recurrence of such pain as she had suffered while in hospital. She was also afraid that she would eventually no longer be able to make her wishes clear. She did not consider palliative sedation an acceptable alternative.

The patient could not yet clearly put into words what her suffering entailed, and she did not wish to die at that point. The independent physician's findings were that the patient would eventually die of her disease. She did not have any specific wish for euthanasia at that time, and that if she was given sufficient palliation there was no reason for her to seek euthanasia. He concluded that the criteria for euthanasia had not yet been fulfilled.

In his November 2005 report the attending physician noted that the patient had clearly deteriorated in the previous month. She was debilitated and looked fatigued. She reported feeling exhausted. Her total dependence and the extreme deterioration in her condition made her feel it was 'all over'. She felt she was being forced to wait for death to come, whereas she would sooner die now. Durogesic was keeping the pain reasonably under control, and her husband gave her occasional injections of morphine. The patient said she could no longer keep up her recent struggle. Now that her condition had clearly got worse – a fact confirmed by the most recent CT scan – and the only prospect was further deterioration, she wanted euthanasia.

The independent physician concluded that the patient was suffering severely from her continuing deterioration. He said he found her suffering (fatigue, complete social deprivation and chronic physical discomfort) to be palpably unbearable. She clearly wished to die as soon as possible.

There were no alternative means, including palliative ones, of alleviating her suffering. The independent physician found that the due care criteria had been fulfilled. The attending physician performed euthanasia by administering 2000 milligrams of thiopental and 20 milligrams of pancuronium intravenously. The committee found that he had acted in accordance with the due care criteria (Regionale toetsingscommissies euthanasie, 2006).

Case 2

As mentioned before, the review committees found in almost all cases that the physician has acted in accordance with the due care criteria. Only in 3 out of 1933 cases were the physicians found not to have met these criteria.

Case 2 is an example of one of the cases where the due care criteria were not met; in this case the problem was that no other physician was consulted.

The attending physician felt he was under a moral obligation to perform euthanasia. The committee found that he had not acted in accordance with the due care criteria.

In 2001 the patient, a 78-year-old man, was diagnosed with a Dukes' C colon carcinoma. He underwent hemicolectomy, followed by radiotherapy. When metastases were found he was given chemotherapy. In 2004 treatment was stopped following the discovery of metastases in the liver. The patient's condition gradually deteriorated, and in December 2004 he discussed the possibility of euthanasia with his physician.

The subject came up again in March and May 2005, and in June the patient made a specific, emphatic request. He had indicated exactly where the limit of suffering lay as far as he was concerned. He always appeared lucid and rational. He did not want to be 'left high and dry'. He had seen relatives suffer for long periods, and he wanted to decide for himself when to die. The patient signed an NVVE euthanasia directive and gave it to the physician, who then indicated that an independent physician would have to be called in. The patient accepted this and said he would talk about it 'when the time came'. In the weeks that followed the situation varied. The tumour grew steadily and the patient dealt with various matters, including his funeral arrangements. In the last week of May 2005 his condition was reasonable. His pain was under control, although he was gradually becoming dehydrated. His physician indicated that there were still some palliative options left. The patient said his suffering was not yet unbearable.

By the beginning of June 2005, however, the pain had become much more severe, and a phone call was made to the attending physician. When he saw the patient it was clear to him that the pain could no longer be controlled. The patient indicated that he had given up the struggle, and asked the physician to perform euthanasia the following week.

The physician recommended that an independent physician would have to be consulted. By then it was 5 o'clock on Friday afternoon and he could not get in touch with a physician trained to give a second opinion in case of a request for euthanasia. He promised the patient that he would call one in on Monday morning. During the weekend a locum prescribed increasing doses of morphine in combination with Dormicum. The attending physician saw the patient again on Monday morning. The patient was very short of breath, had a great deal of bronchial mucus, was restless and unable to communicate, but did respond to pain stimuli. The physician administered 60 milligrams of morphine and 15 milligrams of Dormicum, but the situation remained unchanged. Some hours later he administered 80 milligrams of morphine and 30 milligrams of Dormicum, with no improvement. According to the physician, the patient was now experiencing the kind of suffering he had always been so afraid of. In consultation with the patient's relatives, and despite not having called in an independent physician, the physician decided to perform euthanasia by administering 2 grams of thiopental and 16 milligrams of pancuronium. He felt he was under a moral obligation to do so. He was satisfied that the situation was degrading and unbearable for this particular patient. In his view there was no point in calling in an independent physician now that the patient could no longer communicate.

In an interview with the committee, the physician stated that he had regularly discussed the need to consult an independent physician with the patient. However, the patient had repeatedly postponed the decision, partly because he did not want his wife to have to cope with it. The committee found that, in failing to consult an independent physician, the attending physician had not acted in accordance with the due care criteria. Especially given the length of the patient's illness, the physician could and should have called in an independent physician at an earlier stage. He had remained passive for too long in the patient's wish to postpone the consultation. The committee did not share his view that there was no point in calling in an independent physician now that the patient could no longer communicate. Even in these circumstances, the committee found that the patient could and should have been seen by an independent physician. However, the committee was satisfied that the physician had acted conscientiously in this particular case. It found that he had not acted in accordance with the due care criteria, and referred the matter to the Board of Procurators General and the Health Care Inspectorate (Regionale toetsingscommissies euthanasie, 2006).

The role of physicians and nurses in cases of euthanasia

Nurses have an important role in the stages preceding euthanasia. When a patient discusses the possibility of euthanasia with a nurse, she can try to find out if this patient really wants to end his life or that maybe his request is a 'cry for help' that can be dealt with in another way. Otherwise, she can supply information on euthanasia and explain that only a physician can decide whether or not a euthanasia request will be granted and therefore the request has to be made to the physician. The nurse needs the express consent of the patient to even inform the physician that she talked about the possibility of euthanasia with that patient.

In case relatives bring up the topic of euthanasia, the nurse can explain that only a voluntary and well-considered request from the patient can possibly lead to euthanasia.

If the patient is at home the decision whether or not to grant a euthanasia request is mostly made by the patient's GP in close consultation with the independent physician that has to assess the patient according to the due care criteria. When the patient is admitted to a hospital, nursing home or hospice, physicians are advised to establish a multidisciplinary team. A nurse that is closely associated with the patient (named nurse in the UK) will be a member of this team. This team can advise the physician with regard to decisions to be made. The final decision about whether or not to perform euthanasia is taken by the attending physician.

Nurses can be and often are present when euthanasia is carried out, particularly when the patient is in hospital. They have an important role in supporting the patient and his relatives. The law permits the nurse to assist the physician with the technical aspects of the procedure, but does *not* permit her to administer any euthanasia medication herself. The administration of medication in this context is strictly a medical procedure that cannot be delegated (Besse *et al.*, 2006). It is important to emphasise that anyone who carries out euthanasia and not being a physician will be prosecuted, even if he or she has met the due care criteria.

National and international debate

No consensus in the Netherlands

In the Netherlands, there is an ongoing public debate on the acceptability and regulatory system for medical decision-making concerning the end of life in general and euthanasia in particular. In a study by Rietjens *et al.* (2005) the attitudes of the Dutch general public towards end-of-life decisions in various situations were compared to the attitudes of physicians. Acceptance of euthanasia at the request of a terminally ill cancer patient was higher among the general public (85%) than among physicians (64%). For physicians, acceptance decreased to 11% for a patient without a serious disease. For the general public, this percentage was 37%. One of the determinants of support for euthanasia for the general public was being non-religious. Religious groups are often opposed to euthanasia, mainly on the grounds that no human being has the right to end another person's life. They are of the opinion that this should be left to God or the Almighty.

It can be concluded that, in the Netherlands, there is no consensus of opinion on this. However, a majority of Dutch citizens consider euthanasia acceptable under certain circumstances, such as a terminal illness.

Living wills

There are several types of 'living wills' in the Netherlands, illustrating the point that there is no consensus on euthanasia among Dutch citizens.

An important organisation in support of a free choice on the end of life (including the possibility of euthanasia) is the Right to Die-NL (NVVE). One of the activities of the Right to Die-NL is issuing 'advanced directives' (http://www.nvve.nl/). In this type of living will, the owner asks his physician for a gentle, quick death if a time comes at which there is no expectation of a return to a dignified state of living. The owner of the advanced will document then describes his idea of a dignified state of living. There are many alternative statements for this that may be ticked and signed for. In addition to this there is room for personal statements.

This document solely expresses the *wishes* of the owner. A living will in which the owner states that he would like to die of euthanasia in certain, outlined, circumstances does not guarantee that euthanasia will be performed. There is no such thing as the right to euthanasia, but patients have to go through the process when the time comes. However, this document will make the official side of the process easier, for physicians as well as for patients. A physician can prove, after the death of the patient, that he performed euthanasia at the explicit request of that patient.

One example of an anti-'Right to Die' organisation is the Dutch Association of Patients (NPV). This Association has a biblical/religious background and is opposed to euthanasia. They issue the 'wish-to-live declaration'. Among other things, this type of living will specifies that euthanasia is *not* an option to alleviate suffering for the person who has signed the declaration. Interested readers should refer to Burgerhart (2006).

For Dutch citizens only

Contrary to national and international perceptions, the Right to Die-NL does not prescribe any medication and has no physicians to help people to die. The Right to Die-NL shows people the official path and provides them, on request, with important informative documents. No Dutch physician or institute will ever perform euthanasia or supply deathly medication to visitors from other countries, no matter how serious their conditions might be, or how desperately they 'beg'. For physicians, dealing with requests for euthanasia is very challenging and euthanasia or assisting in suicide is the last thing they want to do, if at all. It may only be when they have an established relationship with the patient, and when they are involved in the entire process of illness and dying, that they might want to consider euthanasia. Only then can they make sure that all due care criteria are met and that they will not be prosecuted. So both from a personal as well as from a judicial point of view, they will never consider requests for euthanasia or assisted suicide from foreign visitors.

Transparency

In the Netherlands the debate on euthanasia is out in the open. The Dutch Government does not turn a blind eye to the fact that euthanasia happens. Only by being completely open about euthanasia is it possible to assess whether physicians who take the exceptional step of terminating a life do so in accordance with standards of due care and quality. Introducing legislation outlining the rules on euthanasia gives anyone requesting euthanasia the strongest possible personal and public guarantee that due care will be taken. By being clear about the standards of due care, and by guaranteeing exemption from prosecution if these standards are met, physicians are encouraged to notify any case of euthanasia.

A high rate of notification sheds light on how euthanasia is being dealt with in practice. This is an important policy goal; in addition to ensuring that due care is taken. It should be noted here that the number of notifications says nothing about physicians' willingness to notify the committees. In order to determine this, the number of notifications has to be compared with the total number of cases of euthanasia and assisted suicide in the Netherlands. A 1998–2002 evaluation of the euthanasia review procedure (van der Wal, 2003) revealed that in 1990, 18% of all cases of euthanasia and assisted suicide were reported and that this figure had risen to 41% by 1995 and to 54% by 2001. In 2005, the percentage of cases reported was approximately 80% (ZonMw, 2007). One of the aims of formalising due care criteria and publishing all the cases that the euthanasia review committees have dealt with is to raise this percentage. As long as not all euthanasia cases are reported there is no guarantee that in all cases the due care criteria are met. Or to put it differently: it might be the case that physicians only report euthanasia when they are fairly sure they have met the criteria and therefore will not be prosecuted. This might explain why in 2005, review committees decided that only 3 out of 1933 cases did not meet the due care criteria. This is also the reason why the Dutch Association of Patients offers the possibility to anyone to report any suspected cases of euthanasia that might be dubious.

It can be concluded that Dutch legislation is no guarantee that euthanasia is always carried out respecting the due care criteria and the duty to notify committees. The main aim of the policy, however, is to bring matters out in the open as much as possible and hence to ensure that maximum care is exercised, while respecting patients' wishes to die.

Euthanasia is well known to occur in many European countries (as well as outside Europe) (van der Heide *et al.*, 2003). If in these countries no legislation is available, and euthanasia is considered a crime, the result is that all cases of euthanasia are 'driven underground' and therefore carried out in secrecy. In this situation there is no possibility at all to assess whether due care has been exercised (Biggs, 2005).

Box 7.2 presents an extract from Dr. Biggs book, as published in *The Observer*, on estimated numbers of 'euthanasia' cases in the UK and other countries, without the practice being legalised. This type of euthanasia is different from that of the Netherlands, but helps to show how, when legalisation is not possible, physicians find other ways of helping patients to die. This is a dangerous position for patients and physicians alike.

Box 7.2 Estimated number of euthanasia cases in the UK

Dr Hazel Biggs, director of medical law at the University of Kent (UK) and author of *Euthanasia: Death with Dignity and the Law*, calculates that at least 18,000 people a year are helped to die by physicians who are treating them for terminal illnesses. Biggs's figures are based on data from countries such as the Netherlands and Australia, which have published research into assisted dying rates, as well as evidence taken from British physicians.

> 'If you extrapolate from countries that have published data, you're looking at quite a large number of patients who may have had their end hastened, not necessarily with their consent,' she said.
>
> 'What this says to me is that we know these practices are going on, but they are completely unregulated. We don't know how many people are volunteers or non-volunteers, and maybe because of that the law ought to be changed so that people can give voluntary consent, which will give them more protection.'

The Observer, 19 September 2004 (see Biggs (2005) for a detailed discussion)

Euthanasia from an ethical perspective

Whether euthanasia is permissible from an ethical point of view depends on the prevailing ethical perspective or paradigm employed by society or governments. Compare for example Consequentialism and Deontology.

Consequential methods of ethics locate the source of moral value in a desirable state of affairs that results as a direct consequence of an action. In this way, Consequentialism emphasises some principle of *the good* as its central tenet. In so far as Consequentialism posits the maximisation of a favourable resulting state of affairs, i.e. some conception of the principle of the good, as its fundamental normative principle, it is opposed to Deontology.

Deontological methods of ethics are generally opposed to Consequentialist methods in so far as they insist that the moral value of an action is wholly independent of the consequences of an action. Deontological methods emphasise duty as the basis of moral value. In this way, Deontological theories emphasise a principle of right action, or *the right*, over the good. Rather than focusing on consequences, Deontologists act according to categorical imperatives. Simply stated these are a set of rules or guidelines that govern their actions, for example: 'you shall not kill'. One of the most important implications of Deontology is that a person's behaviour can be wrong even if it results in the best possible consequences.

It is clear that a Deontologist whose actions are guided by the principle 'you shall not kill' will never think of euthanasia as the right thing to do. From a Consequentialist point of view, euthanasia can be permissible, if (in the given circumstances) death, as a direct consequence of euthanasia, is regarded as a desirable state of affairs by those involved.

Many more ethical approaches can be distinguished, but the two mentioned above are sufficient to illustrate the following point: ethics alone cannot provide the final answer to the question of whether euthanasia is or can be morally acceptable. There is no absolute verdict possible here, as one ethical approach is no better or more justifiable than the other.

Who is entitled to set the ethical paradigm?

If one ethical approach is not superior to the other, the next question is: who is to decide which ethical point of view will be adhered to? This is where the principle of respect for autonomy (Beauchamp and Childress, 1994) can lead the way. Respect for autonomy can be defined as: respecting the decision-making capacities of autonomous persons; enabling individuals to make reasoned informed choices.

The choice that has been made in the Netherlands is to let people decide for themselves whether or not their lives are worth living. As a consequence of that, suicide is not an offence in the Netherlands, whereas it is in some countries. Another consequence is that a person can decide for himself whether euthanasia is an option should that person feel that his suffering is unbearable and without prospect of improvement. People who think of euthanasia as morally unacceptable will not ask for it and as a consequence will not be subjected to euthanasia.

Patients who consider euthanasia morally acceptable often find sufficient peace of mind in the knowledge that euthanasia is an existing possibility. From the evidence presented so far it can be concluded that only a small group of these patients do indeed request euthanasia. Despite the availability of good palliative care in the Netherlands some people regard their suffering as unbearable. Not everybody wants to drink his cup to the last drop. The results of a Dutch study reveal that this seems to be the case irrespective of the level of palliative care that is provided (Georges *et al.*, 2005). To fully appreciate this outcome it should be taken into account that the EAPC Taskforce on The Development of Palliative Care in Europe (2006) has established that the Netherlands is one of the leading countries in Europe when it comes to palliative care-specific resources.

It is not just the patient's autonomy that is being respected; the same principle applies to physicians and other health care professionals, e.g. nurses. Physicians are under no obligation to perform euthanasia and a patient can never compel a physician to perform euthanasia. Physicians have two distinct duties to their patients:

- the first is to relieve suffering, and
- the second is to preserve life

Because honouring a request for euthanasia conflicts with this second duty, physicians are entitled to refuse to perform euthanasia. Nurses may also refuse to assist in performing euthanasia or preparing for it. Neither physicians nor nurses can ever be censured for failing to comply with requests for euthanasia. Dutch law is intended to ensure that physicians and nurses will never have to compromise their personal principles. If a physician refuses to perform euthanasia, then he must refer the patient to another physician who may be willing to grant the request.

Most physicians in the Netherlands are not convinced that palliative care can always alleviate all suffering at the end of life (Georges *et al.*, in press). While Georges may be right in his observation, it also raises several points, including how conversant the physicians are with palliative care, its principles and treatment options. The nature of the relationships that physicians form with their patients, and whether it allows for open discussion and choices, is important. On the other hand, it can be observed that even in the UK, where physicians are known to be very conversant with palliative care, there are patients who express a wish to have their lives terminated (http://www.dignityindying. org.uk/). A study by Ganzini *et al.* (2000) on physician's experiences with the Oregon Death with Dignity Act revealed that substantive palliative interventions lead some – but not all – patients to change their mind about assisted suicide. Ganzini's survey indicates that patients who completed assisted suicide were receiving substantial palliative care, and 81% were in hospice care. It appears that patients do not request assisted suicide because they lack palliative care, but do so even while receiving it. The leading reason for pursuing assisted suicide in this study was fear for loss of independence, and it is not always possible to relieve this fear or the reality of loss of independence (Ganzini *et al.*, 2000).

Physicians who are willing to consider a request for euthanasia feel responsible for relieving suffering when all treatment options have been exhausted. It is crucially important here that physicians are clear and confident that they appreciate the same suffering as subjectively experienced by the patient. These physicians don't want to abandon their patients when they ask for their help and when they may need them most. For them, terminating someone's life through his voluntary and well-considered request, knowing that there is no reasonable alternative, can be an act of beneficence and non-maleficence.

A minority dictating to a majority?

Patients as well as health professionals have different ideas on the permissibility and desirability of euthanasia and assisted suicide. In the Netherlands everybody can act in accordance with his personal point of view about euthanasia. However, in several European countries, where euthanasia or assisted suicide is not a legal possibility, there is evidence (Cohen *et al.*, 2006) that a majority of the population are in favour of legalising these practices. In view of the above, it can be argued that in these countries a minority of the population are dictating the euthanasia paradigm.

In the UK for example, the palliative care lobby, backed by most politicians, the church, the legal system and senior clinicians, have won the day. An amended version of Lord Joffe's Assisted Dying Bill (Joffe, 2006) was heavily debated and stands little chance of becoming law. At the same time, numerous consumer surveys regarding both euthanasia and assisted suicide consistently demonstrate about 80% approval rating for such legislation in the UK (Becker, 2006).

The only possibility for UK citizens who want to die with medical help is to go abroad (e.g. to Switzerland). Only a small proportion of the patients who are willing to pursue this will succeed. Some patients are too weak or too sick to travel and apart from that, not everybody is fortunate enough to have the knowledge and the financial means to make this journey possible. And even those that do might have preferred to die in a familiar environment instead of having to leave their country and home to die. To get an idea of the perspective of patients living in the UK who wish to terminate their lives or who have died with medical assistance by going abroad, readers are referred to 'people's stories' (http://www.dignityindying.org.uk/).

Concluding thoughts

As a starting point, excellent palliative care should always be available for all palliative patients. As palliative care workers, we should do everything we can to understand and make patients' suffering as bearable as possible. However, despite optimal palliative care, there are situations in which people feel their suffering has become unbearable and without prospect of improvement. People's stories (http://www.dignityindying.org.uk/) tell us that this is even the case in the UK, where the quality of palliative care is recognised worldwide as very high. Indeed, for most skilled and experienced palliative care professionals there are limits to what they can do. This is more evident when dealing with a subjective phenomenon like suffering. Since health professionals are human beings, they too have limitations, and therefore cannot always guarantee success in relieving every patient's suffering. We should try as hard as we can, but we should be brave enough to admit that we don't always succeed (de Vocht and Nyatanga, 2007). Taking this perspective, euthanasia is not by definition incompatible with palliative care, but can be seen as a dignified end to good palliative care. The ultimate goal of palliative care is to improve the quality of life of patients and their families. It is therefore imperative to keep the needs and wishes of the patient and his or her loved ones in mind (Janssens and ten Have, 2001).

For some patients, their greatest fear appears to be loss of autonomy, not fear of pain. The standard version of palliative care assures them 'we are going to take care of you', but for these people the real problem is just that: other people taking care of you (Ganzini *et al.*, 2000).

However, it is worth pointing out possible tension here by admitting our limitations or failure to help patients when our sole professional purpose is to care for these patients.

As a logical consequence of the fact that palliative care cannot relieve all suffering, it is not surprising that euthanasia is well known to occur in many European countries as well as outside Europe (van der Heide *et al.*, 2003). Knowing this, it seems clear that there are more advantages than disadvantages to legalising euthanasia and assisted suicide, on the condition that everything possible is done to guarantee that due care criteria are met.

A great advantage is that individual choices can be afforded, both for opponents and advocates of euthanasia, without any health care professional being forced to do anything that his or her conscience would object to. Another advantage is that physicians who are prepared to carry out euthanasia or assisted suicide know exactly what the rules are, and they don't have to be afraid that they will be prosecuted as long as they adhere to these directives.

As euthanasia is out in the open, it is possible to monitor whether health care professionals adhere to these very strict conditions, including the prerequisite that euthanasia can only be carried out at the express request of the patient. The transparency also makes it possible to develop and share knowledge on what procedure to follow when a patient requests euthanasia/assisted suicide and on the most suitable manner to carry it out effectively.

Not legalising euthanasia and assisted suicide seems to lead to a situation where individual choices cannot be afforded (at least not officially) for the majority of the population. As a result, some people die in a way that is not in accordance with their wishes. This may also inadvertently force people who are suffering to go abroad or seek 'back street' solutions. It may drive euthanasia underground, and as a result, make it impossible to monitor these practices at all. Physicians or desperate relatives, prepared to help patients to die, run the risk of being arrested. Equally, physicians may prescribe stronger opiates to end life, which is not the preferred medical way to do this, as this may cause the patient to become delirious. All the same, physicians can still get into trouble if the amount of opiates is not matching the goal of pain control. The lack of knowledge on how to medically perform euthanasia or assisted suicide can result in very undesirable situations, where physicians turn out to be unsuccessful in terminating a patient's life.

Can it be concluded then, in view of the above, that dying with active medical help is an easy thing to do? Does the possibility of euthanasia make it less difficult to die? To be honest I am not convinced this is the case. It is almost always very difficult to face the fact that one is actually dying. Dying does not become any easier because one has the possibility to request euthanasia. Whether to ask for euthanasia or not may well be one of the most difficult decisions a person could make, even in the Netherlands. It takes courage and quite a strong will to do this, particularly when people are really quite ill and have low reserves of energy. Dying is never an easy thing to do and this includes dying at one's own request.

However, the fact that a choice, including the possibility of welcoming or rejecting euthanasia, does exist in the Netherlands, affords justice to the diversity of dying needs found in society. It may be helpful to have a say in the way one wants to die in order to make this highly unique process compatible with one's personal preferences as much as possible. It is also true that despite all the help and choices available, death is an individual 'thing' and the dying person alone has to negotiate the final passage to death.

References

Beauchamp, T. L. and Childress, J. F. (1994) *Principles of Biomedical Ethics*, 4th edn. Oxford University Press, Oxford.

Becker, R. (2006) The moral maze of assisted suicide. *International Journal of Palliative Nursing*, **12**(6), 252.

Besse, T. C., Hesselmann, G. M. and Schuurmans, J. (2006) Richtlijn euthanasie en hulp bij zelfdoding. In: *Palliatieve zorg: richtlijnen voor de praktijk* (eds. A. de Graeff, G. M. Hesselmann, R. J. A. Krol, M. B. Kuyper, E. H. Verhagen and H. Vollaard). VIKC, Utrecht.

Biggs, H. M. (2005) The Assisted Dying for the Terminally Ill Bill 2004: will English law soon allow patients the choice to die? *European Journal of Health Law*, **12**(1), 43–56.

Burgerhart, E. (2006) De NPV-Levenswensverklaring. *Pallium*, April, 28–9.

Cassel, E. J. (1992) The nature of suffering: physical, psychological, social and spiritual aspects. In: *The Hidden Dimension of Illness*: *Human Suffering* (eds. P. Starck and J. Mc Govern). National League for Nursing Press, New York.

Cohen, J., Marcoux, I., Bilsen, J., Deboosere, P., van der Wal, G. and Deliens, L. (2006) European public acceptance of euthanasia: socio-demographic and cultural factors associated with the acceptance of euthanasia in 33 European countries. *Social Science and Medicine*, **63**, 743–56.

de Vocht, H. and Nyatanga, B. (2007) Health professionals' opposition to euthanasia and assisted suicide: a personal view. *International Journal of Palliative Nursing*, **13**(7), 351–5.

European Association of Palliative Care (EAPC) Taskforce on The Development of Palliative Care in Europe (2006) *A Map of Palliative Care Specific Resources in Europe*. http://www.eapcnet.org/download/forTaskforces/DevelopTF-Map.pdf

Ganzini, L., Nelson, H. D., Schmidt, T. A., Kraemer, D. F., Delorit, M. A. and Lee, M. A. (2000) Physicians' experiences with the Oregon Death with Dignity Act. *The New England Journal of Medicine*, **342**(20), 557–63.

Georges, J. J., Onwuteaka-Philipsen, B. D., van der Wal, G., van der Heide, A. and van der Maas, P. J. (2005) Differences between terminally ill cancer patients who died after euthanasia had been performed and terminally ill cancer patients who did not request euthanasia. *Palliative Medicine*, **19**, 578–86.

Georges, J. J., Onwuteaka-Philipsen, B. D., van der Wal, G., van der Heide, A. and van der Maas, P. J. (in press) Physicians' opinions on palliative care and euthanasia in the Netherlands. *Journal of Palliative Medicine*.

Janssens, R. J. P. A. and ten Have, H. A. M. J. (2001) The concept of palliative care in the Netherlands. *Palliative Medicine*, **15**, 481–6.

Joffe, J. (2006) *Assisted Dying for the Terminally Ill Bill*. http://www.publications.parliament.uk/pa/ld200506/ldbills/036/2006036.htm

Koninklijke Nederlandsche Maatschappij ter Bevordering van de Geneeskunst (KNMG) (2005) *KNMG-richtlijn palliatieve sedatie*. http://knmg.artsennet.nl/uri/?uri=AMGATE_6059_100_TICH_R163564411784179

Nyatanga, B. (2001) Cultural issues in death and dying. In: *Why is it So Difficult to Die?* (ed. B. Nyatanga). Quay Books, London.

Nyatanga, B. (2005) The concept of suffering: a hidden phenomenon. In: *Hidden Aspects of Palliative Care* (eds. B. Nyatanga and M. Astley-Pepper). Quay Books, London.

Regionale toetsingscommissies euthanasie (2006) *Annual Report 2005.* http://www.toetsingscommissieseuthanasie.nl/Images/Annuall%20Report%202005%20English_tcm12-2439.pdf

Rietjens, J. A. C., van der Heide, A., Onwuteaka-Philipsen, B. D., van der Maas, P. J. and van der Wal, G. (2005) A comparison of attitudes towards end-of-life decisions: survey among the Dutch general public and physicians. *Social Science and Medicine*, **61**, 1723–32.

Staatscommissie (1985) *Rapport van de Staatscommissie Euthanasie: Deel 1: Advies.* Staatsuitgeverij, Den Haag.

van der Heide, A., Deliens, L., Faisst, K., Nilstun, T., Norup, M., Paci, E., van der Wal, G. and van der Maas, P. J. (2003) End-of-life decision-making in six European countries: descriptive study. *Lancet*, **362**(9381), 345–50.

van der Wal, G. (ed.) (2003) *Medische besluitvorming aan het einde van het leven; de praktijk en de toetsingsprocedure euthanasie.* de Tijdstroom, Utrecht.

ZonMw (2007) *Evaluatie wet toetsing levensbeëindiging op verzoek en hulp bij zelfdoding.* ZonMw, Den Haag.

Web sites

Statistics Netherlands: http://www.cbs.nl/

Dignity in Dying: http://www.dignityindying.org.uk/

Right to Die – NL: http://www.nvve.nl/

Termination of Life on Request and Assisted Suicide (Review Procedures) Act: http://www.nvve.nl/assets/nvve/english/euthlawenglish.pdf

Euthanasia review committees: http://www.toetsingscommissieseuthanasie.nl

CHAPTER 8

Understanding and caring for the dying patient

Brian Nyatanga

Dying is a process that involves, among other factors, disease progression, symptoms deteriorating or new ones appearing, and gradual loss of control and independence by the dying patient. Dying is an individual activity and therefore any care that is going to reflect this individuality must have the patient central. The patient's needs (physical or psycho-emotional) should form the basis on which the delivery and pacing of care is determined. Such care should be based on a sound understanding of the patient and family. This is important because, although the caring professionals may become familiar with death and dying, for the patient, death is a unique experience, which has to be negotiated individually and only once. The other people around the patient can be supportive and sensitive, and this will only help that patient with his or her inner strength in dealing with the final encounter with death. Caring for the dying patient must be seen as also caring for the sum total of that patient's relations (Nyatanga, 1993; Twycross, 1994) including their multitude of emotions. This means seeing the patient as part of a family unit. This unit may include relatives, friends, pets and anyone the patient considers significant, hence the term 'significant others'.

There is a tendency to view the patient with a terminal illness as dying and to forget the positive aspect: that the same patient is in fact still alive until he or she is dead. What we should concentrate on is how to help the patient make the most (if he or she so wishes) in terms of quality of the remaining days, weeks or months of his life. Admittedly, palliative care is about quality, not quantity, of life. A multidisciplinary team approach to such care is therefore a prerequisite for palliative care to succeed, given the complex needs (physical as well as psychological, emotional, spiritual and intellectual) presented by the palliative patient.

Psychological dimensions of the dying

Genuine psychological care is that which affords the patient the opportunity to analyse his own situation. This can be done by the patient asking pertinent questions, from which the answers are used to break down the matrix, in his own mind, about his illness. If this is done properly, the patient achieves more clarity of his own impending death, and this, according to Grey (1996), often leads to greater insights that permit a reintegration of self at a higher level of self-awareness and integrity. It is acknowledged that not all patients can and will ask pertinent questions, but may show signs of anger or any other emotions. In this case the professionals may help the patient 'enter' this psychological analysis by asking open-ended questions, for example 'On top of your illness, what else is making you so angry?'. The assumptions made within the question itself can be denied or nullified by the patient when he chooses his response to your open question. For example the patient may clarify that he is not only angry, but in fact 'livid' about the whole situation he finds himself in. Admittedly open questions allow the patient to select the most appropriate and comfortable response, therefore enabling the analysis of his own situation.

It can be argued that once the dying patient has accepted the reality of his impending death, he may need to withdraw psychologically from the living world. This withdrawal is a gradual process of disengagement (Samarel, 1995) which tends to take place in the last few weeks or days of life. The patient often withdraws into himself for long periods at a time, and this may be seen as removing oneself away from the family and significant others. Disengagement is characterised by progressive lessening of verbalisation by the dying patient, increased sleep even during daytime and not wanting contact with others, including family members. It is not being suggested that disengagement takes place all the time during these last few days, but while in the process, most patients prefer not to be disturbed. It must be arduous for the patient to actively disengage himself from the living world that has been part of his life since birth. It would not be the choice of the patient to disengage, but the realisation that his life is soon to end in a way 'forces' him to engage in this process. This may not be the case with the patient who believes he still has a miraculous chance of 'beating' his illness and go on surviving. However, the actual difficulty in disengaging is that the patient has to have full concentration with minimal external distractions. In order for us (the practitioners/clinicians) to help the patient achieve full concentration, we need to have a fine balance when we prescribe medication that has a potential to impair such concentration while controlling other symptoms. The process of disengagement is emotionally draining for the patient, hence the need to perform it gradually, but often enough so that it remains a continuous aspect of the last few days.

During my experience of caring for dying patients in a hospice setting, I remember hearing a patient shout at her relatives to leave her alone, or in more polite terms 'Not now dear'. One possible explanation for this behaviour can be attributed to the fact that the patient wanted to temporarily shut the world out and continue with disengagement. The fact that she had to shout may suggest a difference or dichotomy in perceptions between the relatives' need to spend more time with the dying patient, and the patient's need for space to disengage. According to Samarel (1995) such misunderstandings often cause distress with relatives who are not obviously aware of what is going on psychologically with the patient. The patient's need for peace and quiet must be explained to the relatives and significant others, but simultaneously taking care that the extreme opposite is avoided. Here the extreme opposite would be that the family, in realising this, may allow too much time apart from the patient, who may in turn perceive this as abandonment. Samarel (1995, p. 101) makes the point that the fear of abandonment is understandable, considering that dying is something that the patient does alone. In this case the role of the professionals would be to facilitate the achievement of a balance by the dying patient between her need for disengagement and not feeling abandoned. It does not seem an easy option at all (if it is an option) to die; hence the view being expressed in this book.

The relatives must be made aware that when a patient has such time, peace and quiet to disengage, what she is basically doing is having a thorough life review. A life review is about putting one's psychological and spiritual house in order. This way of introspection takes time and effort to accomplish. According to Sheldon (1997), this is a time to try to understand the painful things while remembering the successes. The patient may also want to prepare to 'travel' as a whole person (holistically) into the dying mode. This is important because in healthy life, a person's well being is very much dependent on the harmony of all the different dimensions making up that person (psychological, emotional, physical, spiritual, social and intellectual: PEPSSIL). It is therefore equally important that such harmony is also ensured during dying in order to achieve a peaceful and dignified death.

Preserving self-esteem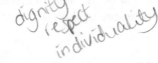

Out of all the fears the dying patient may have, the most frightening is the loss of self-esteem. Loss of self-esteem is often seen as a violation of the very core of personal existence and individual dignity. With this violation follows the loss of control and independence. The dying patient may well understand the need for our nursing care intervention, which, at the same time, by its nature undermines his dignity and assails his sense of privacy. There does not seem to be an easier option in dying. It is well documented and acceptable that nursing care is crucial for the general comfort of the patient, as long as it is delivered in a way that does not make the patient feel less human. One example would be bowel care, which may involve giving suppositories or even performing manual evacuation. This part of care is vital, but before performing such procedures, we should ascertain the patient's previous experiences (if any) and then explain simply why the procedure is necessary. More important is the explanation of how it is going to be done. Arguably most dying patients cooperate fully once they know the 'why' and 'how' of our care intervention.

Patients often feel that they are losing control each time the illness worsens. They may even reject what we, as professionals, perceive as sensible and helpful for them, in favour of what they believe gives them control. For example, they may struggle to the bathroom rather than use a commode by the bedside. Perhaps what professionals should constantly remind themselves is that, for the dying patient, each little bit of control lost is a little bit of ground gained by his illness. This realisation is not easy to accept, particularly for the patient who has always been in control.

Fear of mental isolation

Apart from the observable physical isolation, the dying patient at times feels mentally isolated. There is a propensity by both relatives and professionals to jolly the patient along (Nyatanga, 1993) when he tries to express his fears and knowledge of dying. A patient may express fear of suffocating in his sleep and therefore is afraid to sleep in case he fails to wake up. The same patient may also indicate his awareness of his impending death, and may wish to express his feelings. The patient may feel mentally isolated if he cannot share his fears or thoughts about his dying, and is left to cope alone with his emotions. Allowing a dying patient to voice or articulate his fears often gives the family an opportunity and courage to say 'farewell' or I'm sorry'. Mental isolation is not easy to detect, but might be the most distressing for the patient, and as professionals we need to be aware of this.

Spiritual dimension of care

Unlike psychological care, which is mainly analytical in nature, spiritual care is regarded as that which brings all the component parts (presumably taken apart during analysis) together; hence spiritual care is viewed as a process of synthesis (Grey, 1996). The syncretistic (ability to unite) nature of spiritual care would arguably suggest that it follows after the psychological analysis. The spiritual dimension is concerned with the essence of what it is to be human. Spirituality itself is about how individuals understand the purpose and meaning of their existence within the universe (Woof and Nyatanga, 1998). This encompasses the different aspects of a person's values and beliefs, the meaning of one's existence, relationships with others and one's sense of purpose. As with relationships, Lunn (1993) suggests that these could also be with God or gods or with ourselves. Searching through the literature, including Burnard (1998), Harrison and Burnard (1993) and Smith (1986), it seems that consideration of the spiritual is broadly based on a search for meaning. From a philosophical standpoint this is seen as a search for existential meaning in relation to a given life crisis or event. Death poses a challenge to such personally held belief systems. According to Woof and Nyatanga, some individuals possess a set of beliefs that adequately answer such a challenge, while others may end up suffering as they strive to attain inner peace.

Spirituality is often linked to or associated with religion, but these two are very different in nature (Nyatanga, 1997). It is perhaps those with a faith who may find inner peace through 'talking' to God, Allah or a higher power. What needs explaining is that every one of us has a spiritual dimension but may require different modalities, also known as channels, for dealing with these spiritual needs. For an individual with a faith a religious channel may be most appropriate; hence involving a chaplain or head of that faith may prove successful. For the non-religious individual a different channel is required, and this is often found in someone, something or a power outside that person (King *et al.*, 1994). Religious belief may not always help the dying person. Faith can be severely shaken at times of crisis and questions such as 'How can God let me suffer like this?' are sometimes prevalent, as is the fear of judgement. Stoll (1989) suggests that people may seek sources of strength, a higher power or being for their spiritual needs.

The understanding of the essence of spiritual care has proved difficult as shown in studies cited by Walter (1994). Nurses were found to call in the clergy as a way of dealing with the spiritual needs of their patients. This is disturbing, considering that these studies by Harrison and Waugh were published in 1992, long after nursing had claimed a breakthrough in this area. In view of this, perhaps we need to remind ourselves of the fundamental issues involved with spiritual care.

There are aspects of spirituality, such as genetic makeup, temperament, ethnicity and sexuality, that are inherent within a person, and this is what makes you who you are. On the other hand, there are other aspects that are acquired, such as experience, education, profession, family and even society in which one is brought up, and this makes you what you wish to be or end up being (see also Table 8.1). Therefore different people will have variations in the aspects acquired and hence their sense of purpose may also differ.

However these different people tend to have similar indicators of spiritual health. The following list consists of some of these common indicators.

- Humour
- Hopefulness
- Enthusiasm
- Creativity
- Sharing with others
- Joy
- Ability to flow easily with change
- Finding meaning in struggle and suffering

Suffering is an elusive concept, and readers interested in the medical perspective should consult Cassell (2004). For some philosophical perspectives of this concept, consult Nyatanga (2005).

Aspects of spirituality

The aspects in Table 8.1 are only indicators and should be used as such. For example, if someone was always creative, but does not seem to be so any more, one must question the spiritual well-being of that person. The only problem is that HCPs do not always have knowledge of what this person was like before they became a patient. They often meet them in times of illness, but perhaps speaking to significant others may be a way of gaining this knowledge. Patients who retain all or some of these indicators in their dying may be coping well with their spiritual needs.

Table 8.1 Aspects of spirituality.

Inherent	Acquired
Genetic makeup	Society
Temperament	Education
Ethnicity	Family
Sexuality	Values
Values	Experience
Personality	Profession

It is claimed (Summer, 1998) that patients may experience two levels of spiritual needs, firstly spiritual distress and secondly spiritual despair. A patient in spiritual distress may show signs of mild anxiety, discouragement, anhedonia and unusual questioning of the role and existence of God or a higher power, as well as expressing feelings of guilt and disturbed sleep. Some may even challenge their own belief and value system.

Spiritual despair is characterised by complete loss of hope, with anhedonia leading to refusal to talk to loved ones. The patient may have death wish tendencies, often followed by severe depression. At this point patients can refuse to participate in their own treatment regimen. Spiritual despair is the extreme, which should be avoided if health care professionals can address the patient's needs while he or she is in the spiritual 'distress phase'.

There is the argument that people in spiritual distress will benefit from, among other interventions, unconditional love and non-judgemental approach (Narayanasamy, 1991). A non-judgemental approach assumes that the carer is completely self-aware, and this demands certain understanding by the carer of his feelings and behaviour. It can be argued that self-awareness has two parts that need understanding before we can claim that we are fully self-aware. Each individual has an inner as well as an outer self, and most often will be aware of his inner self in terms feelings, biases, stereotypes, thoughts, beliefs and prejudices (see also Figure 8.1 on the notion of self-awareness). However, he may not always be aware of his outer self, which others see through his behaviour, and may have to rely on feedback from others. It is important to emphasise here that other people will not be aware of his inner feelings, but can only make an interpretation through the observable behaviour. For complete self-awareness the individual will need to receive *honest* feedback on his behaviour in order to reconcile it with his inner self. Once this is achieved it is possible that movement towards a non-judgemental approach is achieved. The emphasis on honesty is made intentionally as it often creates conflict in any polite society such as ours, because we tend to say what we believe others want to hear and obviously cause no harm.

A simple example is when I was living in the nurses' home during my training period and one of the student nurses came into the sitting room wearing her new dress. She asked how she looked, as we were all going out to a party. What was really obvious for us was that the dress did not suit her and secondly she was far too overdressed for this party. However, none of us was honest enough to say so; instead we all commented that she looked wonderful until she had left the room, when everyone was doubled up in laughter. There are so many arguments from this scenario, but the fact is that we did not honestly offer our subjective judgements, which I believe our colleague student was seeking. Some people will argue that it is kinder this way than to upset someone, especially after spending a lot of money on the dress. If this was to be accepted as protecting others then complete self-awareness may never be achieved when it comes to adopting a non-judgemental approach. The dress

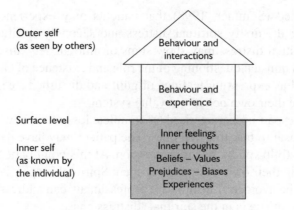

Figure 8.1 The notion of self-awareness.

issue could be seen as trivial, but this behaviour tends to occur as well when the issues encountered are more serious. There are similarities between this notion of self-awareness and that of the Johari Window. For a more elaborate explanation of the Johari Window, see Bayliss (2006).

The notion of self-awareness

A stated principle of palliative care is that it involves:

> The active total care of patients whose disease no longer responds to curative treatment, and for whom the goal must be the best **quality of life** for them and their families. (National Council for Hospice and Palliative Care Services, 1992)

The term 'quality of life' is further explained as focusing on the

Physical
Psychological
Social

and

Spiritual aspects of care.

Actively focusing on the spiritual dimension of care presents a challenge which practitioners often find it difficult to meet. This may be because of a very natural hesitancy about 'not intruding' on what is a very sensitive area at a very sensitive time; or it may be because of anxieties linked to the often indistinct line between religion and spirituality. Yet there is no doubt that the end of life raises issues that inevitably link to spiritual issues – even if these may be rejected – because we are all spiritual beings, even if we are not religious beings or even if we are anti-religion.

Here are a few quotations from practitioners who had had some difficulty in giving spiritual support, but who agreed that without it palliative care could not be said to be holistic:

> I realised that it's not theology they want – it's you.

> It's something you give when you give all of yourself and don't either not respond to questions, as if you haven't heard them, or sort of get into a discussion.

> It doesn't really matter whether you have strong beliefs or none – what matters is actually listening for **and hearing** those needs.

> It's showing them love and recognising their value and worth – until the end.

Looking at the spiritual dimension may be helped by considering the following process.

Based on the work of van Gennep, the notion of bereavement as a *Rite of Passage* is frequently used, but the transition from terminal diagnosis to death may also be seen as a Rite of Passage and it may be helpful to think of it in this way when we try to ensure the inclusion of the spiritual dimension in palliative care.

Once a person realises that his or her illness is terminal, they could be said to be **before the threshold** – that is to say, that there is an understanding that death is imminent. What death 'means' may vary enormously (anxieties about pain; concerns about loved ones; financial worries etc.), but it presents an opportunity for the careful listener to determine what sort of spiritual concerns there may be. The term 'threshold' itself may be a very useful starting point – the person is 'on the verge' of something momentous. Spiritual care at this time may be to do with reconciliation with the diagnosis; with others; with themselves; and – for some people – with God.

Gentle questioning – even something as simple as, 'What do you make of it all?' can be the key to accessing the person's needs. As one patient, previously a palliative carer herself, said, 'We ask about everything else, why do we shy away from that?'.

At the threshold – as death nears the dying person needs to be sustained if she or he is to be able to transcend what is happening. Dying people are, in a very real sense, grieving, and need the same sustaining care we offer to the bereaved. The difference between life (all that makes us who we are) and death comes more acutely into awareness the closer we are to the threshold between the two. As carers, we need to know what the patient sees as a 'good' death and we will not be able to do that unless, when the person was before the threshold, we took time and care to find out, and especially to find out what the spiritual dimension of a 'good' death is for the person.

Past the threshold – after death, the palliative care turns totally to the bereaved. Emotions at this time are often very powerful and rightly need much support. Even so, it is also a time when many questions of a spiritual nature are present. Even those who may have no belief in an afterlife are questioning 'Where is s/he now?' – in the sense that everything that made the deceased who they were has gone – where is it? These and other profound questions, some of which may be religious if the bereaved have a faith, are present in the midst of the loss. Sometimes they are concealed as 'jokes', but careful listening will ensure that we do not neglect the opportunity for expression of fears and concerns.

These three phases could be labelled:

- Pre-liminal
- Liminal
- Post-liminal

and awareness of the different needs at each phase may help us to follow the principle of being *active* in the spiritual care of the dying and so providing truly holistic care.

Spiritual care is about helping the patient to find inner peace, *meaning* in illness and acknowledgement of his pain, often expressed through questions (but not really questions) like 'Why me?'. Such question do not necessarily need to be answered by the carer, but to be viewed as indicators of the patient's need to talk about the impending death. The meaning in question here is what Frankl (1984) sees as the primary motivation in life and not a 'secondary rationalisation'. The meaning is unique and specific to the patient in that it must and can be fulfilled by him alone.

The social dimension of care

Social care recognises that the changes due to life-threatening illness are forcing different individuals to review their roles. For the dying person it means not being able to perform his or her role anymore. This may bring about immobilisation, where shock overwhelms the individual. The dying person realises that there is a mismatch between high expectations or ambitions and the reality of his or her situation. Some people tend to deny this change and may find themselves taking temporary retreat or false competences. While this is happening to the dying person, the same process may be taking place with close relatives. It can be argued that all these reactions are aimed at achieving some kind of equilibrium within the individual, so that proper functioning is resumed as soon as possible. This is where health care professionals can play a leading role in facilitating the achievement of this equilibrium. What we need to bear in mind always is that what seems so logical and straightforward for us may not be that simple for the dying person and his relatives (family unit). Their life is filled with 'chaos' and uncertainty, which may easily lead to conflict, in either a positive or negative way. Understanding of these positive and negative forces may be central to health care professionals in helping the family unit. The whole picture of the family unit needs to be understood in terms of what gaps or roles will be created by the dying person, and who is likely to fill in those gaps. Kurt Lewin talks about analysing the forces involved with any change (Lewin, 1951). Some forces are for the change (hence driving forces) while others are against the change (resistant forces). Before we offer social care it may be worth considering these forces for each family unit. Doing it this way means that we can identify as many negative forces as possible and then prepare ourselves for how these may be turned into positive forces. It also shows us, the carers, at a glance which forces outweigh which, and therefore where to concentrate our energies. Once these forces are identified, they should be ranked as most positive and most negative. Ranking can be done from one to ten.

The following case study is intended to highlight how these forces can be identified and ranked.

Case study

Background history

Pete (46 years old) was in the advanced stages of testicular cancer when the community nurses began to visit him at home. Pete, now divorced from Karen (38), has been living with his partner, Marcus (42), for nearly five years. Since Pete's illness markedly worsened about a year ago, Marcus has been looking after him. Recently, this has become increasingly difficult and stressful for Marcus. As partners they are close and Marcus is overcome by his fears for the likely outcome of Pete's illness and for the loss of their dreams for a life together. Marcus works for a pharmaceutical company and is frequently away from home. Recently, however, due to his concern for Pete, he has started to work from home whenever possible, although his bosses are not sympathetic to his situation. Now Pete needs almost constant care. The emotional stress, worries about his job and the numerous broken nights are taking their toll on Marcus and beginning to affect his health.

Pete is almost entirely dependent upon Marcus for his care and support. He became estranged from his elderly parents, Jim (82) and Martha (76), when they showed themselves unable to accept his relationship with Marcus. Both parents were devastated when, after associating with Marcus for some years, their son had finally left his wife Karen and their two boys to go and live with him. The boys (Dan, aged 14, and Sammy, 9) have continued to see their father at weekends and for holidays. Now, although both boys are fond of Marcus and love their father, they find visiting Pete disturbing and Karen is reluctant to press the matter in such distressing circumstances. The boys miss their outings with their Dad and are deeply upset by his illness, but are unaware of the terminal prognosis. Following her divorce Karen has set the date for her wedding with her new partner, Harvey (34), and is making plans to move away from the area and start a new life. Pete has a younger sister, Marion (44), who married an Australian, Shane (40), when quite young and now lives in Queensland with her twin daughters, Amy and Anne (22). She hasn't been home for some years.

Explanation and analysis

Kurt Lewin (1951) developed a model that can be used to aid understanding of the forces facilitating or inhibiting change. The positive and negative forces for and against change can be identified and their strength subjectively estimated.

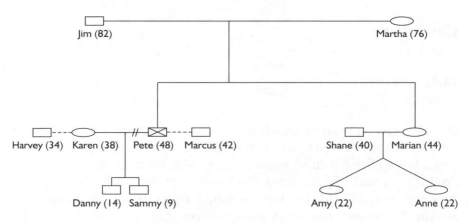

Figure 8.2 Family tree.

An example, given below, provides an assessment relating to Pete's illness. Your own assessment might include other factors or different weightings to those listed here.

An analysis of Figure 8.2 indicates that the negative forces outweigh the positive ones. The pressure on Marcus is intense, despite his desire to continue caring for Pete. It seems possible that either Pete's ex-wife or his sister may be brought in to help. There are concerns for Pete's sons. Dan and Sammy need help now and this may need to increase after their father's death. Professional counselling with a therapist trained in working with bereaved children and young people might be an option. Support and respite for Marcus during these final weeks of Pete's life seems a priority.

The case raises important social issues which you may wish to consider when assessing the needs of the patient and his family. Firstly, the non-traditional pattern of family relationships has occasional exclusions from its membership. For example, Marcus, despite being Pete's partner and primary carer, is not regarded as part of the family. Pete himself has been rejected by his parents. It can be the case that in situations such as this, the family reclaims their homosexual member following his or her death. The partner may be excluded from the funeral or required to sit at the back (Cave, 2000). This is 'disenfranchised grief' a term used to describe grief that is unacknowledged (Parkes, 1996).

Secondly, Marcus may be experiencing 'anticipatory grief' (Lindemann, 1944). *Do you consider that grief can be experienced in advance of an expected death?* If so how might it manifest itself?

Contemporary writers (Parkes, 1975; Fulton and Gotterman, 1980) cast doubt on the idea that grief can be experienced in anticipation of a significant loss. Others take the view that the dying trajectory involves a series of losses for the patient and for those left behind.

Finally, there is the matter of the children's distress over their father's illness and the grief they will experience following his death. The Harvard Child Bereavement Study (Silverman and Worden, 1993) found that children return to their grief time and time again as they reach different stages of their development. Children's understanding of death differs with age. At 14 Dan will have a mature understanding. Sammy, aged 9, will need information and reassurance concerning the changes taking place in his life. Both the boys may need to talk about how they are feeling. There are agencies, such as Winston's Wish, specialising in working with bereaved children.

It must be emphasised that this type of analysis is no different from other types of assessment to elicit patient needs. There is obviously going to be an element of subjectivity within a well-intended objective analysis using such tools; therefore differences are expected. For example, Marcus's care of Pete could also be negative if you felt that he was overprotecting his partner to the extent of denying him his right to information about his sons.

Table 8.2 Analysing the forces created by Pete's illness.

Rank	Positive forces (+ve)	Negative forces (–ve)	Rank
10	The closeness of Pete and Marcus	Pete's dependence on Marcus	10
10	Marcus's care of Pete	Pete's estrangement from his parents	9
6	Possibility of Marion, coming home from Australia to help out?	Pete's worsening illness	9
7	Pete being cared for at home	The strain on Marcus affecting health and work	10
7	Could Pete's ex-wife, Karen, postpone her wedding to help look after Pete?	The boys' distress about their father's illness	10
8	The boys' love for their father	Cost in terms of time, money and relationship for Marion to come back to the UK	7

Table 8.2 shows that negative forces outweigh the positive forces. The interpretation may be that a lot more work is required in order to overcome the negative forces or turn them into positive ones. Marcus carries the brunt of Pete's care. As health care professionals, we must ask certain questions in order to obtain a clearer picture of the situation. For example, how serious is the disagreement between Pete and and his parents? Is it feasible for them to form an alliance before Pete dies? Could they benefit from a mediator to see if the y can end up talking about Pete's deteriorating condition? What other questions can you think of from this case study to help the situation? Once a clearer picture is obtained, specific intervention by health care professionals may be needed to draw the family together and facilitate open discussion. Pete may need additional support in his care to give Marcus a break. The health care professionals also need to concern themselves with Pete and Marcus's wishes. For example, would they like to have their partnership recognised under the civil partnership law? The range of emotions being experienced here may affect the existing family dynamics. It is possible that the end result may be an emotionally closer family or a widening of the present relationships.

Physical dimension of dying

The way in which a patient and the health care professional view the 'dying body' is often the same. However, there may be some differences in perception if the same body is in a lot of pain or discomfort, and the patient, at that time, would view it as a painful immediacy. On the other hand the health care professional may view the same body as an object to be examined or, at the very extreme, as a problem to be solved. This apparent discrepancy has a degrading effect on the patient and can often cause conflict. The way forward would be for health care professionals to share the patient's view about his or her body – hence being on the same 'wavelength' – and then together find a way of intervening.

It is well documented that physical ailments often have a bearing on the psycho-social dimensions of the patient. Therefore health care professionals need to embrace this broad awareness of such causal relationships so that any care provision is as accurate and effective as possible. Some of the most notorious physical complaints of the dying patient include pain, nausea and vomiting, shortness of breath, constipation, noisy breathing due to excessive secretions, fatigue, dry mouth and pressure sores.

Pain

When a patient is in pain it is difficult to concentrate on anything else other than the pain. Pain can be interpreted to mean different things. For example, persistent pain may mean one is incurable or going to die (Twycross, 1997). Such physical pain can often have a bearing on the psychological well-being of a patient; therefore the rule is to consider pain in terms of its totality. This means being aware of the concept of total pain (see Figure 8.3) and also realising that such pain is intertwined and may prove difficult to pin point or separate. It is now well documented (Twycross, 1997) that a patient can experience more than one type of pain at the same time, in which case a comprehensive and multidimensional intervention is called for. This also may require the use of both orthodox as well as complementary approaches to control the pain. In palliative circles the rule is to control pain first and then to manage it. Pain control is achieved by titrating a quick-acting analgesia against the pain. This requires continuous monitoring and adjusting the analgesia according to pain levels until the pain is well controlled. At this point, pain management should start.

Pain management ensures that patients are pain-free all the time as opposed to waiting for pain break through and then offer them pain relief. Admittedly,

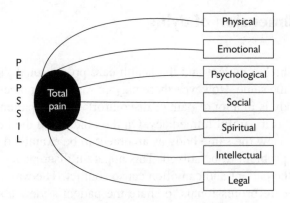

Figure 8.3 The PEPSSIL approach to care.

some patients may wish to experience some of their pain for various reasons. For example, it is possible for patients to attach meaning to their life through the amount of pain they suffer. For some patients experiencing their pain helps to internalise the reality of their terminal illness. Having said this, the point to be emphasised here is that pain management aims to make the patient's pain bearable, that is, something they can live with.

On the other hand if the pain is subsiding due to whatever reason, there is also a need for tapering the opioid analgesia. There is not yet an agreed formula for doing this, but examining the different schools of thought in specialist palliative care, the general rule is to be more cautious. Opioid tapering can safely be achieved by a 25–35% reduction every other day, but still monitoring the patient as usual for any reactions. Some specialist would advocate a 50% reduction every three days. In this case it makes tremendous sense to use the rescue medication while tapering, and the amount given over 24 hours could guide the next dose reduction. All this forms part of the pain management process on top of talking to the patient as well about his pain. It is nonsensical to administer small but frequent doses of morphine, because this does not help the patient's pain, but the prescriber's own fear of morphine. Such mythical ignorance should be laid to rest once and for all. Each prescriber, particularly those not working in palliative care settings, should liaise with more experienced nurses and doctors in palliative care for guidance. I have always found difficulty in understanding those people who know it all, and will not consult with others. While this practice may be trying to 'stamp' one's authority on prescribing, it does not help deal with the pain being suffered by the patient. It is important for all prescribers always to think of the patient first, because ultimately it is the patient who suffers from our mismanagement of his pain.

Nausea and vomiting

Patients may feel nauseous due to several causes, some of which are iatrogenic in nature, for a example as a result of treatment regimes such as chemotherapy. Such iatrogenesis is unfortunate, because the treatment itself is intended to palliate distressing symptoms, yet the side effects may end up being equally distressing, if not worse.

There may be other causes, such as constipation, which can be alleviated by good bowel care approaches followed by bowel management.

Constipation

This symptom can be caused by opioid therapy, morphine in particular. According to Claud and Tempest (1998) clinicians need to understand that the actual need to treat constipation is in itself an indication of failure to prevent it. Constipation should be treated by regular use of laxatives (Lee, 1995) and the laxatives should be titrated until faeces are comfortably soft (Claud and Tempest, 1998). The presence of diarrhoea needs investigation, as this could be an overflow from the underlying constipation.

Dry mouth

This is one of the most uncomfortable symptoms which often causes difficulty when speaking, as the lips often get stuck to the teeth. The use of mouth swabs, frequent sips of cold water and applying vaseline (petroleum jelly) to lips are some of the local measures that will provide some comfort. Pineapple chunks can be useful for stimulating saliva production, therefore lubricating the mouth naturally.

For further detailed reading on the above symptoms, and other distressing symptoms, the reader is referred to the following authors: Claud and Tempest (1998) and Twycross (1997).

The final phase of illness

The person entering the final phase of an illness will often draw from a kaleidoscopic set of experiences, making that person unique. It is from such realisation that each death must be allowed to reflect this uniqueness in its process. The process should be accompanied by its own host of realities which make sense for that person. This may not always be easy to achieve, but it is nonetheless very important that it is afforded the dying person, because life at this stage is one of ever-changing identities from the disease and interactions with others. According to Bertman (1991) the dying person ends up facing a whole range of issues including the following:

- A triangle of interactions between patient and health care professionals and patient and family members.
- The loss of control and independence which often leads to helplessness and hopelessness. This also leads to feelings of worthlessness and low self-esteem.
- The dying process may leave the patient feeling psychologically isolated, lonely, vulnerable, alienated and mutilated.
- The spiritual concerns are brought into sharper focus by scrutinising one's relationship with higher powers and/or God (Nyatanga, 1997; Woof and Nyatanga, 1998). It is here that the dying person examines existential issues, including such aspects as the meaning of life and their sense of purpose in the remaining life.

Thinking and doing all these things does not leave the dying person at liberty to die, but tends to add pressure on him and his relatives to ensure that everything is thought about and thought through properly; hence dying becomes so difficult.

According to Lerner (1978), caring for the dying person can be a blessful encounter although quite ardous. To the dying person the intervention by the health care professionals can be perceived as a real blessing at such a vulnerable time for them.

Concluding thoughts

Understanding the dying person will ensure that death for that person is as peaceful and dignified as can be. The ideal would be to ensure that the harmonious existence of all the holistic dimensions during healthy living is also attained during the dying process. In essence what we are all trying to do as health care professionals is help the dying person through their final passage to death. According to Samarel (1995) all dying people need assistance and this is often apparent in both the verbalisations and non-verbal gestures. The kind of assistance does not always sit comfortably with health care professionals, particularly in the United Kingdom. This assistance should not be miscon-strued as mercy killing, but instead it is assisting through the carers' presence and sensitive support. The dying person should be assisted so that there is a sense of peace even in the presence of physical discomfort. Any discomfort should be minimised and help given in order to put his or her psychological house in order. The health care professional may need to examine her own 'relationship' with death, or as Samarel puts it 'reconcile death in themselves'. It is arguable that to be able to help someone achieve peace, you should be able to have peace in yourself first. To do this effectively may mean to accept death without fear and this has always troubled the human imagination. Fear, if present in the carer, can easily be transmitted to the patient.

Relatives and friends, collectively referred to as the family unit, should be cared for during dying and after the death of their loved one. Health care professionals have a duty to inform them of what may be happening with the dying person and process as well. The family unit needs to know that the dying person will often need to have some time to himself in order to disengage from this life. However, caution must be exercised so that the dying person does not feel abandoned when the family are allowing him that vital space.

Finally health care professionals need to come to terms with their own death first before attempting to help others. Once this is achieved, it becomes quite possible to view patients as living with their dying and not just dying.

References

Ayliss, V. J. (2004) *Counselling Skills in Palliative Care*. Quay Books, Wiltshire.

Bayliss, V. J. (2006) *Clinical Supervision for Palliative Care*. Quay Books, Wiltshire.

Bertman, S. C. (1991) *Facing Death. Images, Insights and Interventions*. Hemisphere Publishing Corporation, New York.

Burnard P. (1998) The last two taboos in community nursing. *Journal of Community Nursing*, **12**(4), 4–5.

Cassell, E. J. (2004) *The Nature of Suffering and the Goals of Medicine*, 2nd edn. Oxford University Press, Oxford.

Cave, D. (2000) Gay and lesbian bereavement. In: *Death, Dying and Bereavement* (eds. D. Dickenson, M. Johnson and J. S. Katz). Open University/Sage, London.

Claud, R. and Tempest, S. (1998) *A Guide to Symptom Relief in Advanced Disease*, 4th edn. Hochland and Hochland, Cheshire.

Frankl, V. E. (1984) *Man's Search for Meaning*. Simon & Schuster, New York.

Fulton, R. and Gottesman, D. J. (1980) Anticipatory grief: a psychosocial concept reconsidered. *British Journal of Psychiatry*, **137**, 45–54.

Grey, R. (1996) The psychospiritual care matrix: a new paradigm for hospice care giving. *American Journal of Hospice and Palliative Care*, July/August, 19–25.

Harrison, J. and Burnard, P. (1993) *Spirituality and Nursing Practice*. Avebury, Aldershot.

King, M., Speck, P. and Thomas, A. (1994) Spiritual and religious beliefs in acute illness – is this a feasible area of study? *Social Sciences and Medicine*, **38**, 631–6.

Lee, E. (1995) *A Good Death*. Rosendale Press, London.

Lerner, G. (1978) A death of one's own. In: *Facing Death. Images, Insights and Interventions* (ed. S. Bertman). Hemisphere, New York.

Lewin, K. (1951) *Field Theory in Social Science*. Harper & Row, New York.

Lindemann, E. (1944) Symptomatology and management of acute grief. *American Journal of Psychiatry*, **101**, 141–8.

Lunn, L. (1993) Spiritual concerns in palliative care. In: *The Management of Terminal Malignant Disease* (eds. C. Saunders and N. Sykes). Edward Arnold, London.

Narayanasamy, B. (1991) *Spiritual Care, A Resource Guide*. Quay Publishing, Wiltshire.

Nyatanga, B. (1993) Emotional pain in palliative care. *Palliative Care Today*, **II**(III).

Nyatanga, B. (1997) Cultural issues in palliative care. *International Journal of Palliative Nursing*, **3**(4), 203–8.

Nyatanga, B. (2005) The concept of suffering: a hidden phenomenon. In: *Hidden Aspects of Palliative Care* (eds. B. Nyatanga and M. Astley-Pepper). Quay Books, Wiltshire.

Parkes, C. M. (1975) Determinants of grief following bereavement. *Omega*, **6**, 303–3.

Parkes, C. M. (1996) *Bereavement: Studies of Grief in Adult Life*, 3rd edn. Penguin/ Harmondsworth/Routledge, London.

Samarel, N. (1995) The dying process. In: *Dying; Facing the Facts* (eds. H. Wass and R. A. Neimeyer). Taylor & Francis, Washington.

Sheldon, F. (1997) *Psychosocial Palliative Care. Good Practice in the Care of the Dying and Bereaved*. Stanley Thornes, Cheltenham.

Silverman, P. R. and Worden, J. W. (1993) Children's reactions to the death of a parent. In *Handbook of Bereavement; Theory, Research and Intervention* (eds. M. S. Stoebe, W. Stroebe and R. O. Hansson). Cambridge University Press, New York.

Smith, R. (1986) Toward a secular humanistic psychology. *Journal of Humanistic Psychology*, **26**(1), 7–26.

Stoll, R. (1989) The essence of spirituality. In: *Spiritual Dimensions of Nursing Practice* (ed. V. B. Carson). W. B. Saunders, Philadelphia.

Summer, C. H. (1998) Recognizing and responding to spiritual distress. *American Journal of Nursing*, **98**(1), 26–31.

Twycross, R. (1994) *Introducing Palliative Care*. Radcliffe Medical Press, Oxford.

Twycross, R. (1997) *Symptom Management in Advanced Cancer* 2nd edn. Radcliffe Medical Press, Oxford.

Walter, T. (1994) *The Revival of Death*. Routledge, London.

Woof, R. and Nyatanga, B. (1998) Adapting to death, dying and bereavement. In: *Handbook of Palliative Care* (eds. C. Faul, Y. Carter and R. Woof). Blackwell Science, Oxford.

CHAPTER 9

Cultural issues in death and dying

Brian Nyatanga

Introduction

One would speculate that dying is much easier in some cultures than in others. If that was the case, one would then further speculate on the differences in those cultures, and what it is that makes dying easier. However, considering the discussion in Chapter 7 of legalised euthanasia in the Netherlands, such speculation may be limited, as death is an individual thing. The understanding of different cultural needs is important when caring for dying patients. An individual's cultural background influences their way of behaviour and view of the world they live in. In Britain today 5.5% of the population is from minority cultural groups. This chapter argues that cultures in a plural society like Britain are not static but are continually changing. The nature of this change is discussed by looking at the processes of enculturation and acculturation. It is also argued that although some cultural change may take place, some basic rituals at birth, death and dying remain unaffected. This then raises the need for health care professionals to be aware of the original (purist) value and belief system of each individual patient's culture (that is, before acculturation) and hold that as a broad framework while assessing the current values and beliefs of that individual patient.

The difference between culture and religion is briefly discussed, before selecting a few cultural groups to discuss their beliefs and practices during dying and at death. This is important because the basic tenet of palliative care (which is largely caring for dying people) is to view and treat the patient holistically. To this end this chapter aims to provide the reader with practical information about caring for the various cultural groups.

If we are to meet the needs of all our patients in palliative care, then we need to appreciate their varying cultural backgrounds. There is a need for us to understand their expectations during death and dying and how they grieve.

This chapter intends to raise awareness about the different cultures in our society and so appreciate the challenges facing all health care professionals.

Before examining the specific cultural issues in death and dying it is important to consider the nature of the cultural changes in today's society.

When providing palliative care to any patient, it is very important that the carer has an idea of the patient's value and belief system. This is even more important in today's Britain, which has over the years shifted from being mainly Christian to becoming a more plural society. This shift is also true of other societies around the world. In Britain, the National Council for Hospice and Specialist Care Services (NCHPCS) has indeed recognised the importance of understanding the cultural backgrounds of patients in terms of health. The Council (1996) has now published a report on the need for greater involvement by members of the ethnic minorities in palliative care. The Council calls for measures that would improve access to hospices and specialist palliative care services by all minority cultural groups to be put into practice. While this may seem an encouraging report, it places enormous demands on all health care professionals and other agencies, particularly those in palliative care, to have an increased understanding of the needs of these different cultural groups during death and dying. It must also be emphasised here that there are differences within the same group of people; for example, just as the English have sub-cultures within them, so too do Muslims and Jews.

Throughout this chapter an attempt will be made to give you information which can be readily used in your clinical settings. It will focus on the different cultural beliefs found in this country, highlighting their needs and rituals during dying and at death. This is important, as death rituals and funeral rites are arguably the final stage of reconstituting the bond between the deceased and the bereaved. However, it is not possible to cover every culture in depth; therefore an overview of the beliefs and care of the dying and bereavement will be provided.

As stated earlier, it is important that we consider the nature of the changing cultures in today's Britain and consider the implications this may have for the care we provide during dying and after death.

The nature of the changing cultures

The dynamic nature of cultural change is a global phenomenon. In order to appreciate this concept I should start by offering one definition of culture, as suggested by Devito (1992). Culture may be defined as:

> a relatively specialised life-style of a group of people, consisting of their values, beliefs, artefacts, ways of behaviour, and communication

This is a sociological definition which suggests that our life is strongly affected and influenced by our culture. Our cultural background influences the way in which we view the world and how to behave in it in relation to other people. Any group of people living together tend to produce their own language, laws and mode of thinking as a distinguishing feature from others.

From the above definition, it is implied that culture is transmitted from one generation to the next – a process known as **enculturation**. In other words, culture is something that is learned and not inherited. For example a Roman Catholic bishop is not born to be celibate, but learns from the teaching of the church and then takes the vow of chastity which subsequently influences his life. Children learn their values from parents, society, peer groups, school and other similar institutions. When you look at today's Britain, with its multitude of cultures, it is evident that the original process of enculturation will inevitably undergo constant change through interacting with other minor or smaller cultures. In any society, the original culture of any group will be influenced and changed according to its exposure to the media, schools, institutions, communities and even direct contacts. The result is often a modification in the original culture, either for survival or because they now share, to some extent, the values and beliefs being offered by the other influence. This process is known as **acculturation** (Devito, 1992) and can be witnessed when the smaller cultural groups, such as immigrant ethnic minorities, modify their culture in line with the host culture. It can be argued that the host culture also changes (although to a small extent) as it understands the minority cultures within it.

If we accept that acculturation exists in any plural society, we cannot therefore afford, as health care professionals, to hold stereotyped views about any given culture. To do so would make us rigid, unrealistic and denying people's individuality, and as a result would increase the assumptions about the cultural group(s) in question. To assume as Twycross (2003) puts in terms of pain control, is to make 'an ASS of U and ME '

In a plural society, the original (purist) cultural forms are regularly challenged and someone's impending death will bring these philosophical questions into sharper focus for the individual. Perhaps what we ought to do is hold a framework of each cultural group and how they would behave in their original (purist) form, that is before acculturation, and then assess each individual patient to determine their present value/belief system. It is on the above premise that the information contained in this chapter is based.

It should be emphasised at this point that, some cultures will be resistant to change and will therefore defend traditional practices, which often results in inter-cultural conflict. For example an immigrant family may not modify its values and beliefs even after years of exposure to the host culture. It has been

claimed (Devito, 1992) that open-minded and young people tend to be accul-
turated more easily than the older generation. It has been suggested (O'Neill,
1995) that even after considerable acculturation, most cultures still retain their
rituals and practices at birth, marriage and during death and dying.

Culture vs. religion

In some cases, culture and religion may have strong associations, but they
are two different entities. It is, however, possible to find people's lives being
influenced by both their culture and religion (faith). It is also true to say that
some people's religion (faith) forms the basis of their life and hence becomes a
way of life, often referred to as a paradigm. For example, if there were a need
to change the way of this basis of their life, the change itself could often be
seen as a paradigm shift. In difficult times people derive strength and inspiration from their religion, as may be seen from this comment: 'My strong faith
helped me through my problems'.

On the other hand, people who do not believe in a god (atheists) or agnostics
(those who believe in silence on the topic of god because it is such an abstract
concept) still have a culture and spiritual needs that influence their lives. As
stated above, culture includes the values and belief system of individuals. In
view of these differences, what may be plausible is to ensure genuine inter-
cultural and religious communication. This should enable people of different
values, beliefs and ways of behaving to work collectively for the common goal
and, in this case, the dying patient.

If we are to understand the needs of the patient and family, then it is also
imperative that we start by understanding ourselves and how our preconceived
ideas and beliefs may prejudice our perceptions of other cultures. This forms
the basis of palliative care philosophy and the provision of culturally sensitive
services (Sheldon, 1995). Within the palliative care philosophy are the principles of acceptance and of believing the patient, who may have practices unlike
our own, unconditionally. The focus of care shifts from curative to predominantly caring. Caring is about improving the quality of life by blending our
competence (skills) with compassion. Maintaining this blend is important in
today's health care provision, where resources are depleted, thereby threatening to erode the fundamental core of caring for the dying patient and family.

The following information is from a selection of different cultures and will
focus on the traditional beliefs and care of the dying and bereaved. For detailed
accounts of these, the reader is referred to Rees (1997), Neuberger (1994a) and
other books listed at the end of the chapter.

Judaism

Main Beliefs

As far back as the 6th century BC the members of the tribe of Judah have been known as Jews. Jews believe in only one God, who they believe created the Universe (Green, 1993). They place a very high value on the family and also observe the Ten Commandments of the Old Testament of the Bible. This makes them practise charity and tolerance towards other people. Although they all believe in the Jewish Holy Book – Torah – which is made up of the first five books of the Old Testament, there is now a wide diversity of religious practices among the Jewish community.

Care of the dying and bereaved.

According to Neuberger (1999) the Jews would do anything in their power to preserve life, since they believe it a special gift from God. They expect the same conviction from health care professionals and doctors in particular, as they are believed to be God-sent. Being God-sent, the doctor is expected to have the healing powers and should never say the end is imminent (Neuberger, 1994a). In view of the way in which Jews see the doctor as having God's power to heal, there is a potential conflict of expectations, as the doctor should not see him- or herself as having these powers, thereby placing medicine in a predicament, not just with the patient but other professionals like nurses.

Jews would expect the dying patient to still continue to eat and drink, which again highlights how difficult it is for them to accept death. Neuberger (1999) sees this behaviour as highlighting the strength of their passion for life. It may be an acceptable aim for most of us in palliative care to achieve a comfortable and dignified death for all the patients we care for, but this concept of a 'good death' is foreign to traditional Jewish thinking. It therefore goes without saying that health care professionals need to be sensitive to such issues and establish the patient's prevailing beliefs about their dying.

It is customary for a dying Jew to have psalms recited, and they should not be left alone. Jews believe that if you leave a dying person alone he will die more quickly. They are against anyone removing cushions or pillows from under the head, as this will again hasten death. This has implications for health care professionals in terms of pressure area care and other nursing procedures that involve moving the patient. It is here that automatic pressure relieving aids would be satisfactory and culturally acceptable. If the patient has to be moved in the case of incontinence, clear explanations should be given before the procedure is undertaken.

Once the person has eventually died, the body should be left alone for about 10 minutes. A Jewish tradition of placing a feather over the mouth and nose to observe for signs of breathing may be followed. This is a way of ensuring that death has definitely occurred before any organs (if needed for donation) can be removed for possible transplants. It is tradition that the eyes of the deceased should be closed by one of their children.

Burial should take place within 24 hours and should only be delayed by the Sabbath (their holy day of prayer and rest). Strictly, Sabbath commences at sunset Friday and ends at sunset Saturday.

A Jewish burial usually involves throwing large quantities of earth onto the coffin using spades in a definitive noisy manner. This is to emphasise the reality of the death to the bereaved and also signals the beginning of bereavement. This is then followed by seven days of mourning (Shiv'a) with prayers at home every evening. The next phase is 30 days of less mourning (shloshim) with prayers at the synagogue. After this, there is a period of eleven months' rest before the consecration of the tombstone.

It is the Jewish tradition to 'hang on' to life for as long as possible and to ritualise death fully as a way of going through bereavement. Care within palliative care should permit Jews to follow their rituals by creating a conducive environment that shows understanding and sensitive to their needs.

Islam

Main beliefs

Islam means submission to God, and is the religion practised by Muslims. Muslims believe in Mecca, their religious centre, and every Muslim has a religious obligation to visit Mecca in Saudi Arabia at some point in their life time. After this visit, Muslim men no longer shave their beard, and they have an outward sign of their maturity. They also wear headgear (a topi) as a sign of respect. In public Muslim women cover their heads all the time with a special cloth, as a form of cultural respect.

Muslims believe they have five duties to perform according to the teaching of Mohammed the Prophet.

- Faith (Shahada): declaring their allegiance to God.
- Prayer five times a day facing Mecca.

- Alms-giving (zakah): donating to charity. Using the British pound sterling as an example, Muslims will donate to charity £2.50 for every £100 savings they have.
- Fasting for 30 days (Ramadan).
- Making a pilgrimage to Mecca (Hajj).

Unlike Jews, Muslims believe death to be God's will. Once they realise they are dying, they may wish to die at home, believing hospitals are irrelevant at this point. They see hospitals as places you go to be cured.

Care of the dying and bereaved

Traditionally a Muslim patient may wish to sit or lie facing Mecca, which is to the south-east of the UK. According to leading Muslims, a relative will usually whisper a call to prayer in the patient's ear and then family members will recite prayers round the patient's bed. If no relatives are available, then any practising Muslim can call to prayer and help to give the patient religious comfort.

After death, the body should not be touched by non-Muslims. The head should be turned towards the right shoulder, as Muslims believe this will enable the deceased to face Mecca at burial. The body is not traditionally washed nor are the hair and nails cut. The body should be fully covered (from head to toe) by a white sheet. Burial is usually within 24 hours and Muslims do not practice cremation. Muslims believe that the dead person will be asked religious questions about their faith and how they lived their life and that the coffin should be deep enough to allow the dead person to sit up while answering such questions. It is thought cremation would not allow this important procedure to occur.

Few Muslims believe that their bodies ought to be buried in the country in which they were born, such as India or Pakistan.

Hinduism

Main beliefs

Hindus believe in different gods and goddesses, who are all manifestations of one god in different forms. They do not believe in a standard way of worship; therefore some may meditate quietly while others go to the temple once or twice a week. Hinduism is the religion of the vast majority of the Indian people. Hindus believe that what an individual does with their life in this world affects what will happen to them in the next world (a belief known as karma). Hindus are also vegetarians because they do not believe in killing animals for food. The cow is a sacred animal, a symbol of gentleness and unselfish love.

Caring for the dying and bereaved

Most Hindus would prefer to die at home, where they will receive readings and hymns from the Hindu holy book (the Bhagavat Gita). Some Hindu patients may wish to lie on the floor, a symbol of their closeness to Mother Earth (Rees, 1997, Chapter 2). A Hindu priest should be called to perform holy rites.

After death the family usually washes the body at home. If in hospital and the relatives are not available, the nursing staff can wash the body, but should obtain permission first. Disposable gloves should be worn by staff and the body wrapped in a plain sheet without any religious emblem.

Hindus prefer jewellery, sacred threads and other religious objects on the body not to be removed.

The priest may tie a thread around the neck and wrist of the dying person as a blessing (Rees, 1997). It is traditional for the priest to sprinkle holy water from the River Ganges over the dying person's body. The priest may also place a sacred Tulsi leaf in the patient's mouth.

Sikhism

Main beliefs

Sikhism was founded by Guru Nanak, who according to Brennand (1992) tried to combine the best of Hinduism and Islam. It was Guru Nanak Dev who also first gave women equal rights more than 500 years ago, but today's society (Sikh) is reluctant to honour these rights. Sikhism originated from the Punjab region in India. Sikhs believe in one God and it is the responsibility of each Sikh to form their own relationship with God. It follows that each member will have their own way of worshipping. Sikhs believe in re-birth, which will eventually achieve ultimate understanding through a unity with God. They also believe in equality of all people irrespective of colour, caste or creed. The faith of the Sikh is symbolised by 5 'K's:

- **Kesh**: uncut hair
- **Kangha**: wooden comb
- **Kara**: iron wrist band

- **Kirpan**: short sword
- **Kachha**: short trousers

Sikhs believe in reading from their holy book – Guru Granth Sahib (Adi Granth), through which they receive spiritual guidance.

Care of the dying and bereaved

A dying Sikh may receive comfort from reciting hymns from the Granth Sahib. If the patient is too ill to recite himself, then relatives or a reader from the Gurdwara (Sikh temple) can do so instead.

After death the body can be touched by non-Sikhs, but the family may wish to wash the body as part of the rites before laying it out. The 5 'K's should not be removed from the body, with the hair not trimmed and head covered.

Sikhs value a calm peaceful expression on the face of the deceased, as the face will be displayed to those paying their last respects before burial takes place. The body should be covered in a plain sheet with no religious emblem. Sikhs are always cremated, except for stillbirths who may be buried.

Buddhism

Main beliefs

Buddhist faith centres on the Buddha, who is revered not as God, but as a leading example of a way of life. It has been suggested that Buddhism is a paradigm based on the belief that by destroying greed and hatred humans can attain perfect enlightenment. It is believed that greed, hatred and delusion cause suffering to mankind. Traditionally Buddhists take responsibility for their lives and believe that their actions on this earth will be judged in a subsequent life. It is therefore important for a Buddhist to behave properly and this includes a strong belief in the sanctity of life. As a result of this conviction Buddhists condemn abortion and active euthanasia.

Care of the dying and bereaved

Care of the dying will differ among various Buddhist groups, but the most important and common consideration is the state of mind at time of death. A Buddhist will want to die with a 'clear mind', free from sedation, as this has an effect on the character of rebirth. This has implications for health care professionals on the use of drugs that may jeopardise this mental clarity. Clinical experience suggests that most Buddhists are reluctant to take analgesics, especially opioids, as they believe that any sedation is problematic. There is scope in considering 'informational care' that is giving honest information to the patient, and the use of complementary therapies such as acupuncture for pain control.

Buddhists believe that peace and quiet are imperative at death, as this has a bearing on the character of rebirth. They also need peace and quiet for meditation and some seek counselling from fellow Buddhists. Chanting may be used to influence the calmness of the mind.

When a Buddhist dies it is important that a minister or monk (of the same group) is informed as soon as possible. The usual time between death and burial ranges between three and seven days, depending on the relevant Buddhist group. Most Buddhists prefer cremation to burial.

Christianity

Main beliefs

The belief in Christianity back dates some 2000 years when Jesus was born in Bethlehem into a Jewish family. Christianity is the religion of those who are followers of Jesus. Christianity is divided into different groups and the reader is reminded that the common denominator is the belief in Jesus Christ, the Holy son of God. Christians believe they can approach God through his son Jesus Christ. According to the teaching of their holy book (the Bible), Jesus is the result of a virgin birth (a concept that is perceived emphatically by some Christians, while others appear more pragmatic about the truth of this theory). Christians believe in Jesus as the Messiah, and a saviour of the universe. *Christos* is Greek for *Messiah*, hence the name Jesus Christ.

All Christians believe in an afterlife, either in heaven or hell. Heaven (often described as paradise, see Luke 23:43 in the Bible) is the place where those who have followed God's commandments[1] will go for eternity. Hell is the opposite of heaven, where all sinners (those who have not followed God's teachings) would go and be burnt subject to eternal torment. Most Christians, when approaching death, will continually assess themselves and how they feel they have lived their lives on this earth, and their chances of a new life after

---

1 Readers who are not familiar with the commandments are referred to Exodus 20:1–17 in the Old Testament of the Bible).

death. It is quite common for those whose faith in God is ailing to rediscover it as death approaches. Arguably this is also true of other cultures and religions. However, there are cultural differences in the way Christians in different countries view death (Neuberger, 1994b). For example, Christians like Roman Catholics and Protestants in Ireland are much more open and celebrate death, whereas their counterparts in Britain would not be as open or be celebrating death (Neuberger 19994c). In Britain, death appears to be still viewed as a taboo topic, not because of the pain and loss caused, but perhaps because of fear of the unknown. From this, death is seen as a source of denial and potential enslavement of the dying and their family. Although attempts have been made by those who believe in 'near death experiences' to explain what happens after death, it still remains the biggest source of fear and uncertainty.

Rastafarian

Main beliefs

Rastafarianism originated from the West Indies – Jamaica and the Dominican Republic in particular. Rastafarians are descendants of the slave trade families who were forced out of Africa to work in the sugar and other plantations. The Rastafarian movement was first established to strengthen the resistance to slavery, and emphasis is placed on identifying with mother Africa. A central component of Rastafarian belief is the accession of Ras (Prince) Tafari as the Emperor of Ethiopia in 1930. They believe that the Emperor is a divine human being, the Messiah of the human race who will lead all black people to freedom. Rastafarians respect the Old and New Testaments as scriptures, but do not consider themselves as Christians (Green, 1993). However, they believe that God's spirit has been reborn in Ras Tafari. Rastafarians believe they are the true Jews and that they will eventually be redeemed through repatriation to Africa, which they believe to be their true home and Heaven on earth. Rastafarians do not believe in organised worship and there is no clergy, but the belief centres on a deep love of God. Rastafarians believe that the Temple of God is within each individual member's body, which should therefore be kept holy.

Care of the dying and bereaved

Rastafarians are reluctant to undergo any treatment that may contaminate God's Temple (their body) and therefore Western-style treatments may come second to alternative therapies such as herbalism. Blood transfusion and organ transplants will not be acceptable. Orthodox members of the Rastafarians show their symbol of faith and black pride through their dreadlocks hairstyle, which is not cut at all. After death Rastafarians have a 10-day period of reading the scriptures. Prayers are said in the name of Ras Tafari, the new Messiah.

Paganism

Main beliefs

Paganism is a religious belief centred and maintained orally as opposed to having a Bible (Talmud). Although Pagans have different practices within paganism, they seem to have some common fundamental principles.

Firstly, they have a belief in a Goddess, which forms the initial focus for their worship. This is the feminine principle. The Goddess has different names (maiden, mother and crone), which when translated represent youth, maturity and death respectively (Prout, 1992).

Secondly, Pagans believe in exercising their capabilities and abilities but without causing harm to anyone. This is the principle of freedom with responsibility. Most Pagans believe in their closeness to nature, and are therefore prone to adopt alternative lifestyles.

Thirdly, Pagans believe that they have no control over what happens in their life. This is the principle of destiny. Although this may seem to present a possible conflict with their second belief, this does not in any way negate their responsibility, but perhaps provides a basis for coming to terms with death and dying.

Finally, Pagans believe in the recycling of energy after death. This equates with their belief in reincarnation. The recycling of energy is their way of feeding energy back to the Earth, but usually this is thought to happen through burial as opposed to cremation.

Caring for the dying and bereaved

Pagans would prefer to die at home where they will be able to prepare positively for death. Pagans have their own spiritual advisors whom they expect to visit even when in hospital. A hospital chaplain would not be acceptable unless specifically requested. A dying Pagan may request privacy to worship with friends and family. In hospitals this request may be made during visiting hours.

Pagans would be prepared to donate their organs and would receive transplants and transfusions. According to Prout (1992), following death last offices may be carried out by nursing staff and with no special rituals. Bedside prayers will not be acceptable after death, but can be performed by fellow Pagans just before death. Pagans are in most cases buried, and ideally they prefer a fellow Pagan to conduct the funeral service.

Readers who are interested in pursuing the cultural issues in palliative care are referred to the following authors: Burja (1983), Cowles (1996), Haroon-Iqbal *et al*. (1995) and Jonker (1996).

Final comment

When all these groups discussed above are being cared for, particularly during death and dying, there are some patients who may not speak or understand the English language. Although health care professionals have tried to find interpreters, one concern with the Asian community is using a family member as an interpreter. There is a catalogue of ethical as well as personal dilemmas in such practice. Most Asian people believe that the diagnosis of cancer carries a stigma; therefore the person with a diagnosis would like to maintain his or her own privacy about this. Thus asking a family member to interpret leaves the patient's 'secret' exposed, therefore denying him his privacy. The patient will often find that his family members become curious about the extent of the illness and the likely prognosis. Most of the family members used as interpreters are the younger ones who can speak both languages, and the role often burdens this young person with emotionally charged information. It is not as if he or she can detach himself or herself from the patient afterwards, like health care professionals can when they go off duty. This young interpreter has to go home with the patient, who in this case could be his father, mother or uncle. What ends up happening is that the patient will not go back to the hospital for his next appointment. The family member who is the interpreter feels distressed and is often torn between helping his family and self-protection. One solution might be for the hospitals and hospices to hire the services of professional interpreters who will work alongside specialists in palliative care. This arrangement might also encourage the members of the Asian and ethnic minorities to access the palliative care services, or any hospital service.

Palliative care on the whole should continue to be sensitive to the unique needs of patients from the ethnic minority communities (Oliviere, 1999) in order to provide high-quality care.

Concluding thoughts

Throughout this chapter a broad framework has been applied for most cultural groups in Britain today. Within this framework emphasis has been placed on the kaleidoscopic nature of cultures under enculturation and acculturation. The main point to emerge is that cultures within a plural society undergo changes and thus it is important to assess each individual's cultural needs while holding this broad framework. It is vitally important that as carers we should hold principles that value people's cultural choices and permit their beliefs to flourish even when they approach death. This understanding should be demonstrated in the way we assess patients' cultural, spiritual and religious needs. More often than not, on admission to our care, agnostics end up giving Church of England (C/E) as their religion, just because the way in which we ask questions implies that they should have a religion. Unless we are aware of the cultural differences and adept in our skills of assessing, it is possible that the cultural and spiritual needs of most patients will not be identified accurately. In palliative care we are looking after the whole person (holistic care) and during the terminal phase, cultural and spiritual needs are often elevated and more prominent.

It is very reassuring for any patient to have their care personalised (e.g. recognising a birthday). Acknowledging the festival of Ramadan to a Muslim confers respect. This can have many advantages including the following:

- Demonstrating to the different cultural and religious groups an understanding of their varying needs, thereby reassuring them in order to gain their trust.
- Raising awareness amongst carers and thereby increasing access to hospitals and hospices by different cultural (ethnic minority) groups.

Perhaps this attitude shift may counter the ever-increasing allegations that hospitals, along with other public institutions and their staff, do very little to understand the needs of the different cultural groups in this country. This is clearly not the case within palliative care, but if we do not actively show that our care is 'culture deep' we risk being tainted with the same accusations.

It should be the aim of every palliative care setting to provide and guarantee, through various ways, *'palliative care for all'*.

Additional information on handling funeral arrangements

Transporting a body for a funeral abroad

If after death the family wish to send the body back to its country of origin, certain requirements should be satisfied. Steps must be taken to arrange this, but the funeral directors will and should in practice arrange almost everything.

The following should be taken as guidelines only. Note that the fees quoted are likely to differ regionally or have increased since writing this chapter, in line with other market forces.

The family of the deceased must:

1. Contact the funeral director of their choice and inform him of their wish to send the body abroad.
2. Register the death (normal procedure), but inform the registrar that the body is to be transported abroad.
   - Instead of issuing the usual certificate of disposal, the registrar will make a copy of the death certificate for the family to give to the funeral director. There is usually a small charge.

The funeral director should do the rest of the following:

1. Apply to the coroner for an 'out of England' order, usually granted within a day or two.
2. Supply the airline carrying the body with a 'Freedom from Infection Certificate', usually obtained from the doctor who signed the death certificate. The doctor may charge a fee varying from virtually nothing to £15.00. (The airline may refuse to carry a body that suffered from an infectious disease.)
3. Provide a zinc-lined coffin which must be hermetically sealed (airtight).
4. Provide a certificate to prove that the body has been embalmed.
   Some countries require a Consular seal from the relevant embassy.

All arrangements can be completed in a matter of days. The cost varies (often by as much as £300.00) since different airlines have different freight charges.

NB: If the body was the subject of a coroner's inquest and the verdict was death by natural causes, there are no problems and the above procedure can be followed. If the death was unnatural, for example murder, drug overdose or poisoning, then the repatriation will not be allowed until the court case is over. In this case the body will be held in the city mortuary until proceedings are complete. In this case practitioners need to consider the implications for relatives, especially those who wish to perform rituals as soon as possible after death.

References

Brennand, J. A. (1992) Funeral rites in multi-racial society. *Unpublished Research Project*, University of Sheffield.

DeVito, J. (1992) *The Interpersonal Communication Book*, 6th edn. HarperCollins, New York.

Green, J. (1993) *Death with Dignity. Meeting the Spiritual Needs of Patients in a Multi-cultural Society*. Nursing Times Publications, London.

National Council for Hospice and Specialist Palliative Care Services (1995). *A Statement of Definitions*. Occasional Paper 8: Specialist Palliative Care. NCHSPCS, London.

Neuberger, J. (1994a) *Caring for Dying People of Different Faiths*. Wolfe, London.

Neuberger, J. (1994b) A Jewish perspective on palliative care. *Palliative Care Today*, **3**(3), 32–3.

Neuberger, J. (1994c) Cultural issues in palliative care. In: *The Oxford Textbook of Palliative Medicine* (eds. D. Doyle, G. Hanks, N. I. Cherny and K. Calman). Oxford University Press, Oxford.

Neuberger, J. (1999) Judaism and palliative care. *European Journal of Palliative Care*, **6**(5), 166–8.

Oliviere, D. (1999) Culture and ethnicity. *European Journal of Palliative Care*, **6**(2), 53–6.

O'Neill, A. (1995) Cultural issues in palliative care. *European Journal of Palliative Care*, **2**(3), 127–31.

Prout, C. (1992) Paganism. *Nursing Times*, **88**(33), 42–3.

Rees, D. (1997) *Death and Bereavement. The Psychological, Religious and Cultural Interfaces*. Whurr, London.

Sheldon, F. (1995) Will the doors open? Multicultural issues in palliative care (editorial). *Palliative Medicine* **9**(2), 89–90.

Twycross R. (2003) *Introducing Palliative Care*, 4th edn. Radcliffe Medical Press, Oxford.

Further reading

Burja, J. (1983) *Cultural and Social Diversity: A Third World in the Making*. Open University Press, Milton Keynes.

Cowles, K. V. (1996) Cultural perspective of grief: an expanded concept analysis. *Journal of Advanced Nursing*, **23**(2), 287–94.

Haroon-Iqbal, H., Field, D., Parker, H. and Iqbal, Z. (1995) Palliative care services for ethnic groups in Leicester. *International Journal of Palliative Nursing*, **1**(2), 114–16.

Jonker, G. (1996) The knife's edge: Muslim burial in the diaspora. *Mortality*, **1**(1), 27–43.

CHAPTER 10

Funerals: functional or dysfunctional for the bereaved?

Brian Nyatanga

Introduction

Funerals are triggered when a death occurs. The nature of the funeral and rituals surrounding it depends on the beliefs held by the deceased (initially), the family and society at large. In addition to the existing information in this chapter, I intend to refer to the concept of death discussed earlier and how this may influence funeral rituals. In funerary terms, death becomes a measure of life, while at the same time, life becomes transparent against the background of death. Death evokes all sorts of reactions and behaviours in us all, and in a way it is a catalyst that, when put into contact with different cultures, precipitates the central beliefs and concerns of a people. It can be argued that death is the removal of the most precious thing (life) from this world. This has often attracted comments like 'timely' or 'untimely', and has also influenced how the bereaved express their emotions. In a way. funerals are the most immediate reflective 'vehicle' of remembering the dead. Such remembrance can be positive but in some cases it is tainted with sadness, feelings of loneliness, emptiness and negative thoughts, or may even be disruptive. As will be explored in detail later, funerals can be celebratory occasions, while in other cases they can be sad and painful events.

It may be worthwhile to look briefly at the sociology of death and dying. This will help to put into perspective the role(s) of the funeral. For the reader who wishes to explore the sociology of death in more depth, the following sources are recommended: Seale (1998), Clark (1996), Prior (1989) and Sudnow (1967).

Death is often compared to the Sun (which provides the source of life in the natural order) in that it provides the central force or dynamism underlying life and the structure of the social order. Death is influential in religious circles, philosophies, arts, political ideologies and medical advances. On the other hand death sells newspapers (depending on who has died and also how the death occurred) and may be used as a way of ascertaining the adequacy of social life. Death is used to sell insurance policies, and this is a thriving business which has now developed different policies for different types of death – for example accidental death insurance policy. Death is often used as a basis for comparisons of different cultures and societies, using life expectancy as an indicator of social progress, decline or even stasis.

The role of funerals

One evening my 14-year-old son, now 22 (during our regular chats) tried to wrestle with the 'what happens after death' notion and why people react in different ways to a death. He thought that some people feel very angry about someone's death, while on the other hand others may celebrate the life of that person. These are obviously ways of coping or dealing with life without the person who is now dead. The anger may be triggered by the fact death has 'robbed' this person of his life, and in all cases without agreeing or consulting on how and when death should occur.

From an anthropological perspective death has received social recognition through various processes and activities including funeral rites and rituals. Such ritualistic activities have, arguably, one common purpose, and that is the disposition of the dead body. One often wonders why most people and of different cultures find it necessary to have some kind of ceremony for this disposition? Would it not be acceptable or suffice for a family to dispose of the body quietly without a funeral or any ritualistic practice? Firstly, death should not be seen as an incident affecting the individual and his immediate family (Denison, 1999), but as having significance for the wider community. The community will therefore take part in celebrating the life lived by the deceased and ensure a decent and dignified disposal of the body. The method of disposing of the dead body should adhere to specific contexts and characteristic of the deceased person's value system. For example a Christian (e.g. Roman Catholic) context will be different from an Islamic context of disposing of the body. Denison argues that in the Christian context, for example, the words said during disposition are shaped by the theological motivation of that faith, and may not be appreciated by a group with a different faith.

Leming and Dickinson (1998) argue that funerals and their rituals allow individuals of every culture to maintain relations with ancestors. It is obvious that not everybody believes in ancestral practices, but funerals still play a part after death. This suggests that there are other reasons of significance. Funerals have a potential for uniting family members by physically bringing them together and also allow for shared expression of emotions, leading to further solidarity. This view is also supported by Bee (1994) who claims that apart from weddings, funerals tend to bring a large gathering of people together, some related and others through friendship or acquaintance.

However, it is also true to say that disagreements also emerge, particularly over the 'how the funeral should be conducted' aspect (Walter, 1997). This often leaves some family members not satisfied with the ritual. When a ritual is performed, the intended outcome is to regain control by the immediate family and community over the disruptiveness caused by death. With control comes the repositioning of the bereaved in order to establish a new meaning for their lives without the deceased.

On a wider scale, funerals are thought to reinforce social status, fostering group cohesiveness and ultimately perpetuating the social structure of a society. Following on from this, there is also the argument that society cares for its people in health and illness, and through funerals and ritualistic practices the emotional well-being of the bereaved is promoted. If this is the case it follows that funerals have no benefit for the deceased directly or otherwise, but are perhaps there to benefit the bereaved and the community. Bayliss (1996) argues that the bereaved do not gain financially from a death, since funerals are themselves a costly business, and may create an ordeal even where the deceased was not closely attached to those left behind. Perhaps one example is the national outpourings of grief witnessed after the deaths of Diana, Princess of Wales, Martin Luther King and President John F. Kennedy. The question Bayliss poses, which is worth consideration, is why we have developed a custom which sometimes causes more distress at an already vulnerable time? This makes dying more difficult, particularly if the dying person is constantly being reminded of the complexity and cost of funerals. Here cost should be viewed not only in terms of finance, but also in emotional and physical terms (human cost).

However, since there is arguably an increased tendency for the living to organise their own funerals, it would be interesting to explore whether this eases their dying. One positive outcome of this pre-arrangement might be the benefit to the bereaved in that they do not have to organise the funeral. On the other, one argument might be that by pre-arranging the funeral, the bereaved might be deprived of the only most immediate therapeutic 'exercise' to perform following the death of their loved one.

Another role played by funerals is put forward by Malinowski (1984) who claims that funerary rituals play a significant role in opposing or counteracting the centrifugal forces of fear, helplessness and dismay that often follow after death. In following such rituals, it helps to rebuild the family's weakened solidarity and rejuvenate any shaken morale. This is often achieved through reflection and or reminiscence.

Some of the things that such rituals tend to reflect on, are the good or positive aspects of the deceased, while ignoring the negatives. For example, each time I have attended a funeral ceremony, rarely have I heard of any demeaning accounts made about the deceased, even when it was obvious that during the deceased's lifetime there was hardly anything positive to applaud. Durkheim (1954) argues that funeral rituals are intended as a collective expression of sentiment, therefore anything negative would not help the emotional well-being of the bereaved. Another argument put forward is by Fulton (1995) who claims that funeral rituals help to incorporate the deceased into 'the world of the dead'. Therefore, helping the deceased to enter to this world requires a recall of all the positive aspects of the deceased to be highlighted. By going through the actual process of funerals, it also signifies the end of life and the separation of the dead from the living (Fulton, 1995). Such argument may only be temporary and viewed mainly in physical terms, as it can be argued that some deceased people tend to continue to maintain some kind of relationship or contact with their bereaved relatives. This will be explored later under the heading 'Living with the dead', but for now the focus moves to how funerals can be different in their functions; hence the need to classify them.

According to Mandelbaum (1959) there are two main types of funerary function: manifest and latent.

The manifest funerals are those associated with mortuary rites that are readily apparent, including disposal of the body, helping the bereaved practically and financially, public acknowledgement of the death and demonstration of continued group and family solidarity.

The latent funerals are to do with funeral customs that include economic and reciprocal social obligations that are re-enacted at the time of death. They may include restrictions and obligations placed on family members with regard to attire, demeanour, what they eat or drink and social etiquette. Mandelbaum claims that this is important to show family support and togetherness. It is still common practice in most Western cultures to wear black attire to a funeral. Therefore, arguably, black is seen as synonymous with sadness, a sombre mood and generally that something is not right. For example the word *black* was used to describe the British Government's 'Black Wednesday' under Prime Minister John Major and Chancellor Norman Lamont. The association of black with bad or negative experiences does not help black people, or our quest as a nation to view death as a natural process of life and help to eradicate the taboo of death. What may be plausible would be a change to a brighter colour, which might convey a change in mood and perception of death and allow a celebration of life.

It must be pointed out at this stage that funerals and their ritualistic practices are not the invention of the developed *Homo sapiens* or those in the Western world. Fulton (1995) claims that funerals existed well before 3000 BC and it is believed that Ancient Egypt had its funerals around the same time.

Living with the dead

It can be argued that the deceased do not really leave us entirely, despite the assertion made above that they enter the world of the dead. The deceased tend to play different and numerous roles in the lives of those still alive. For example, the dead may continue to exercise control over the living by stipulations left in their wills. It is quite common for the dying person to rewrite his will from the death bed in hospital, hospice, nursing home or even his own home. While the intention is largely to leave the dying person's house in order, it also adds an extra dimension for him to consider at a most vulnerable time. Wills often create a point of tension and conflict among the dying person's family, especially if the family members do not receive what they believe to be their legitimate share. This belief is often based on several things, including the following:

- How close the member was to the deceased
- Caring input given during the illness (usually where the illness is chronic)
- Relationship to the deceased, e.g. wife, son, daughter or close friend
- The overall value of the estate of the deceased

One of the key points to emerge from this is how dying may produce other pressures apart from those emanating from the illness itself; hence dying can be extremely difficult for the dying person and those left behind.

The process of living with the dead can also be seen from the legacy left through his or her memories, which often take a strong hold on the affairs of the living. Memory is a passion no less powerful or pervasive than love. It prevents the past from fading away. On a non-physical level, the dead person is almost always present with the living. This is arguably because he is too meaningful or precious to the bereaved to be forgotten. One view is that the deceased tend to give the living direction and in some cases a purpose to enjoy life once again. According to Bertman (1979) there is another view which suggests that we need the dead to release us from obligations, open up new potential and give us a sense of belonging and strength to carry on with our lives. Such is the essence of symbolic immortality. Kolakowski (1983) views, on a large scale, the memory of the deceased as having an inspirational effect on the living to the extent that they (the living) have made magnificent creations such as the Taj Mahal, the Egyptian pyramids and other monuments. It is therefore plausible to accept and suggest that such memories of the dead help us to bring about continuity and meaning to our existence. This goes a long way in explaining why different Governments (despite the different political ideologies) maintain national cemeteries for their fallen soldiers.

Western society also encourages the creation of memorial funds, such as that of Diana, Princess of Wales and more recently that of Stephen Lawrence, a black teenager who was the victim of racist murder in South London. Such memorials serve two main purposes:

- The dead continue to live with the living and not to be forgotten
- Lessons are learned from such a death (Stephen Lawrence) and from this a better future for all is guaranteed by improving race relations. Lessons can also be learnt from what the dead person stood for and believed in (e.g. Diana and her numerous campaigns, including banning landmines). Although these deaths may have strong influences on how authorities will act in future in terms of introducing new laws, such laws alone may not be enough to change the hearts or attitudes of all people. Attitudes, as discussed in Chapter 1 can only be affected, and may take a long time to change or shift.

In some instances statues of particular influential individuals are erected as a way of keeping the dead in 'touch' with the living. However, history confirms that not everyone believes in the immortality of the spirit (Kolakowski, 1983) and the Russian Communists are a perfect example when they decided to embalm the remains of Lenin.

This non-belief in the immortality of the spirit creates another dimension of our relationship with the dead. Memories of the dead can also invoke fears in the living. One view is that if the dead are not properly appeased through *acceptable* rituals then their 'ghost' will create mayhem with the living. The belief in the existence of ghosts was seen by Frazer (1968) as a human belief in the immortality of the soul. This belief is passed down from race to race and generation after generation. What tends to happen here is that the living sacrifice their real 'wants' in life in favour of the imaginary 'wants' of the dead. It is from this perception that possible explanations can be ascribed to the different ritualistic behaviours witnessed worldwide. In my home country, I have witnessed some tribes appeasing their dead by pouring home-brewed beer over the grave and dancing and ululating all night long. Such a ritual may not sit comfortably with a middle class family in England; hence the use of the term 'acceptable'. Instead, flowers may be the acceptable ritual, although looking back in time, flowers were traditionally used to conceal the smell of the dead body until burial took place. In today's society, where there are technological advances to prevent the dead body from smelling, there has been a considerable shift from flowers and now some people are opting for money or donations instead.

It was important to explore the above as a way of trying to put into context some of the basis for funeral rituals witnessed in different families, cultures and societies at large.

Remembering the dead through obituaries

One method of remembering the dead found in funerary rituals is the use of obituaries. When obituaries were first introduced at the beginning of the 18th century, their main aim was to act as funeral notices for the whole community (Leming and Dickinson, 1998), thereby inviting all community people to come and pay their last respects to the dead person. With this historical function in mind, it seems that obituaries today have shifted in their aim in favour of different agendas. For example, in the United Kingdom, it is not always abundantly clear why and for whom obituaries are written. Proponents of obituaries would argue that they are written for the wider community to inform them of the death (often viewed in the context of loss) of one of their members. The context of loss here is taken to mean that the community has lost the contribution of the dead person; hence it is death that has deprived the community of the continued contribution. It is claimed that obituaries also help to place the bereaved in sharper focus for the whole community to appreciate their grief, and where possible to offer emotional as well as practical support. Therefore it is logical to argue that obituaries provide a therapeutic value for the bereaved.

When you read obituaries it becomes obvious that they are not part of everyone's funeral ritual, regardless of culture or other individual differences, but for a selected few. When you read obituaries it is plausible to think that those individuals who have made personal and significant contributions to the social order of their community are afforded this rather prestigious biographical summation. In other words, such summations may also offer a platform for the assessment of the meaning of life by the bereaved and the immediate community. However, what makes this assertion less persuasive is the fact that not everyone who has made such contributions receives a biographical summation of their achievements. Over the years, obituaries have revealed that not a lot of women or black and minority ethnic people feature in them, leaving Long (1987) to conclude that obituaries are a characteristic of the middle class white male. Obituaries were also viewed by Gerbner as 'social registers' for the middle class. But let us not be myopic too quickly here; perhaps the middle class white male was the one who made the contributions to the community worthy of mentioning. It is therefore only right that their bereaved should benefit from the therapeutic effect that obituaries supposedly provide.

The contrary view is that history confirms that women and black and minority ethnic people have also made significant contributions to the social order of their communities, but have received very little if any mention. It is interesting to note that where obituaries for women or ethnic minorities appear, they are almost always relatively shorter than those of middle class white men. It is always going to be *machtpolitik* to argue that the length of the obituary is a reflection of the degree of significance of the contribution to the community by the deceased. It may also not be surprising to find that the 'judges' of the values of such contributions emanate from the same middle class background. It is clear that the poor, regardless of their contributions, may not always be afforded such glamorous summations; therefore the 'poor man's' obituary could be said to be the actual funeral itself and verses printed in local newspapers, often selected from a book.

While obituaries may remain narrowly focused on the middle class population, perhaps they could include additional information on how the contributions have actually impacted the lives of others. Such information might act as a point of emulation by the present generation while ensuring continuity within the communities. This may be one attraction in death: to know that one would leave a legacy of memories to help the living.

Funerals: functional or dysfunctional?

There are arguments on both sides to suggest that funerals are capable of being functional as well as being dysfunctional, and this is true across different cultures. It is argued (Mandelbaum, 1959) that participating in the funeral ceremony of a loved one affords the bereaved a sense of belonging to a larger social community. A funeral offers a platform to express painful emotions in a safe and supportive environment of the social community. During a funeral, it is quite acceptable to cry publicly while trying to come to terms with life without the deceased. Many authors, including Van Gennep (1961) and Mandelbaum (1959) agree that a funeral is a 'rite of passage' which marks, for the bereaved, the end of life and real separation of the dead from the living. It is from Van Gennep's work that more understanding of the rite of passage is drawn. Van Gennep claims that any ritual that involves passage usually moves from one state to another in a tripartite manner.

This trilogy involves:

1. **Separation**: the deceased individual is removed from his or her previously held social position or role. For example, the dead person is separated from the living.

2. **Transition**: the deceased individual is moving between the previous social state and a new one, and here the individual is excluded physically and also in a symbolic way from society. It is here that the dead are believed to move away from the world of the living.

3. **Incorporation**: the deceased individual is reintegrated into a new social order. For example a new social order may be to incorporate the deceased person into the 'world of the dead'. It can be argued that incorporation is most commonly facilitated by various funeral rituals, and we have all probably witnessed or heard of deaths where the body has not been recovered and most relatives will not rest until they have performed their rituals with the body.

Looking at Van Gennep's findings, it may seem persuasive to be simplistic and to suggest that in such rituals there is a beginning, a middle and an end. However, the real point to emerge, and which should be emphasised here in terms of funerary rituals, is that it is the middle part (transition), that takes centre stage and is mainly focused on during death and bereavement. One speculative assertion would be to believe that funeral rites could help to ease the transition phase for the bereaved; hence it is imperative to have a funeral. This is a time often characterised by intense emotions, disbelief and a desire to come to terms with what is happening. Littlewood (1993) claims that many researchers now believe that there is real potential in such speculation being accurate, but more work needs to be carried out following Van Gennep's initial thesis.

What may also need researching is whether the length of each transition has any bearing or effect on the overall benefit to the bereaved. In any inquiry of this nature cultural variations should be taken into account.

On the other side of this argument is the fact that funerals and their rituals are potentially dysfunctional. There is one argument that suggests that funerals become dysfunctional if they do not change or modify in line with changes of the modern world. The values, whether therapeutic or otherwise, placed upon funerals by our ancestors could not possibly remain static in the face of the changing political and socio-cultural orientations of the modern world.

Funerals can be dysfunctional if, for example, the cause of death was not natural, such as in the case of death caused by terrorist bombing, murder or assassination by another person. It is possible and has happened before (Fulton, 1995) that such funerals have also caused the death of others through the emotional turmoil created by the first death. Revenge killing may also cost lives and thousands of pounds in destroyed buildings and other possessions. It is now believed that the after-effects of violent deaths (relived through funerals) can lead to physical pathological symptoms (Sheatsley and Feldman, 1964), such as headache, upset stomach and tiredness. There is a tendency to be preoccupied with the death, feeling dizzy and numb. There is an exception to this in that some murders or assassinations (for example that of Martin Luther King) can result in functional funeral rituals, because the mourners try to propagate and bind the philosophy of the deceased; in this case, that of non-violence (Fulton, 1995). Such funerals are often seen as opportunities to make a real statement and to uphold the philosophy, contrary to expectations of retaliation. Finally, it is important to consider the different levels of our social organisation and acknowledge that one funeral can be functional at one level of social life such as the community, but may not be so at a national level. It is important to argue that every funeral ritual should serve a purpose, but the question that needs to be clarified is: what purpose?

Funeral directing

There is another dimension to funerals in particular in the changing world of business and modernisation. In most developed countries death has become institutionalised. This is witnessed when the disposal of the dead body is done by 'strangers'. The bereaved find themselves paying an undertaker to transport and dispose of the body of their loved one. The undertaker and other workers in this line of work are providing a service which has grown so rapidly that it necessitated a change of name from Undertaker to Funeral Director. The funeral director has an industry which is charged with a significant function with dead people and their families. This dramaturgical function of handling the deceased's body while caring for the emotions of the relatives creates a need for a director to ensure a fine balance between the business affairs of the organisation and the bereaved people's emotions. Rees (1997) claims that the funeral directors and their employees receive professional education and the Association of Funeral Directors sets examinations for the employees to take. This can only be a positive way of ensuring that the bereaved are treated professionally and sensitively at a time of distress.

Funeral directing seems to be a thriving business for several reasons, the most obvious of which is the increased number of people dying. One other reason is that the funeral director and his service function in communities that are no longer as cohesive and where neighbourhood support is now nonexistent. Most developed world families are now depleted due to working away from home and other demands; therefore the funeral director may be the only person available to offer (at a minimal charge) support and comfort to the bereaved. Another possible reason is the death-denying attitude of Western societies, with the UK leading the list, which in turn prevents important decisions from being made until death has occurred. The bereaved would therefore not have prepared themselves for the funerary arrangements, including 'window shopping' for prices of coffins and other relevant requirements. There are other services which, with close scrutiny, the bereaved may not require, but end up buying them all in a package as provided by the funeral director. This view sounds as if funeral directors are not regulated, but this is simplistic, because today's public are more knowledgeable (therefore question more) and the funeral directors will be keen to be seen to be ethical in their practices. Most funeral services perform a remarkable function, but there are a few pockets of the service which take advantage of those in the throes of grief.

As an example of a caring service, the funeral director arranges (with permission from the bereaved) for the reconstruction of the dead body through embalming, which is arguably the cornerstone of this industry. It is argued that, for the bereaved, embalming makes viewing of the body and paying of last respects a much more 'palatable' experience. This is the time the bereaved are thought to 'store' the last picture and memory of the deceased, with which to live the remainder of their lives.

It is here that perhaps health care professionals can play an influential role by providing relevant literature on funeral services as part of the information given to the relatives of a dying patient. It is not uncommon for relatives to ask for details of funeral directors and services from the professional carers. We therefore have a duty to assist the bereaved, particularly at a time when their emotions may cloud their judgement. It can be argued that for the bereaved to make the best possible choice of funeral service they need information and education. They need information about all the options available and the prices. The bereaved need to be assured that it is quite OK to shop around for the best service and price. The cost of a funeral will vary according to the choice of coffin, whether it is a cremation or burial, the number and type of cars required (e.g. limousine/hearse) payments for the minister, church and doctor's certificate (if the body is to be cremated) and additional costs for catering if required. The bereaved may also benefit from knowing the different prices for a range of coffins, and at the end of this chapter a range of coffins is shown, including the costs. The cost in brackets is based on 2007 prices, and the other list is the 2001 prices. As can be seen, the choice of coffins is wide and varied and tends to cater for everyone's financial position.

The information given later in the chapter shows the general funeral services and the cost implication depends on the type of coffin ordered. The costs are based on current prices in the United Kingdom, which are also subject to change in line with inflation and other factors. The bereaved should be able to compare the cost of the whole package and not just a single item. Some of the services are optional, such as flowers.

Children and funerals

The decision as to whether or not a child should attend a funeral can be fraught. Discussion can range from pointing out that when a pet dies it is often given an elaborate 'funeral', so why when a grandparent dies are children excluded?, to a view that children should not be subjected to what may be a highly charged emotional experience at such a young age. It is not possible to be dogmatic, as much may depend upon the nature of the child's attachment to the deceased, but bearing in mind the efficacy of ritual in assisting with grief, it is important to consider what excluding a child might mean, and to examine whether not permitting children to attend a funeral has something to do with adult fears and concerns, rather than with the child's needs.

Funeral directors suggest that the important thing is to ascertain what the *child* wants, and if the wish is to attend, to make sure that as much information about what will happen is given first. Children will often follow the model of the adults around them, and this can be a good opportunity to learn healthy grieving practices. Children who, for whatever reason, do not attend the funeral of someone close to them can still feel included if, for example a poem they have written or a picture they have drawn is included as part of the ritual.

It may be useful to remember (Jackson, 1978):

> Children have a lot of life to live, so it is important to guide them in such a way that they develop wise and healthful attitudes towards their feeling, their lives, **and their deaths**.

General information on a funeral service

The average cost of a funeral service will be about £1375. This cost will include initial consultations, paperwork and overheads. The cost will increase to £1705 if two limousines are required.

Transportation: This will include moving the body to the funeral director's premises and placing the final disposition. Provision of a hearse will cost £120 £132, and a limousine will be £99. Excess mileage, that is over and above 20 miles, will be charged at £1.00 per extra mile.

Care of the body: This will include embalming and dressing the body – £50.

Facilities: This includes the cost of viewing, funeral or memorial ceremony if it is held at the funeral premises. Normally there is no charge for viewing the body, even outside normal working hours. Use of the chapel for overnight vigil will cost £110. There is a surcharge of £160, for Saturday and Sunday, for using a funeral director and up to four of the staff.

Optional facilities: These include flowers, music and obituary notices, and if the director pays a third party to do a job, this cost is added. Flowers can range from (£20) for the sympathy basket to (£350) for the superior coffin cluster. It is helpful to find out whether there are any other charges, often listed under 'miscellaneous'. Once a fuller picture of the service and cost is obtained the bereaved are arguably in a better position to make a decision.

The use of coffins and casket will have varying costs; for example, the Regent casket will cost £2750 while the basic Glen coffin will cost £330. While it is important to know about these varying costs, what is more important and should be communicated to the bereaved is that the amount spent on a funeral does not necessarily reflect how much you loved the person who has just died. The key factor is sensibility and affordability.

Table 10.1 Coffin types and prices.

Name	Description	Cost
The Glen	Sapele mahogany effect – white taffeta interior (WTI)	£330
The Consort	Gloss teak effect – white tafetta interior	£429
The County	Gloss walnut effect with engraved panels – WTI	£500
The Herald	Light gloss oak effect with decorative panels single raised panel lid – WTI	£588
The Priory	Satin finished oak veneer, antique brass finished handles – white quilted satin interior	£610
The Balmoral	Gloss finished oak veneer, moulded panel lid solid wood handles with antiqued brass fittings – white quilted satin interior	£644
The Cathedral	Gloss finished mahogany veneer, engraved panels distinctive solid wood handles and pewter finished fittings – white quilted satin interior	£698
The Traditional	Solid oak timber, traditional design, double panel raised lid – antique metal handles, embellished satin interior with extra deep fill	£896
The Opal	Solid oak construction, high gloss dark oak finish – six antique bronze finished cast metal handles – satin interior	£1017

There is also a range of high-quality caskets constructed in either steel or solid timber and the cost may range from £735.00 for the Sentinel casket to £2,500.00 for the top of the range, the Regent casket.

Concluding thoughts

Throughout this chapter some of the roles and functions of funerals and their rituals have been discussed. The funeral rituals tend to differ according to the cultural background of the bereaved family and therefore will have differing meanings. However, the funerary practices witnessed in different cultures all serve a similar purpose, that of disposing of the body of the deceased. The rituals performed signify a variety of things, such as a celebration of the deceased's life, bidding farewell to the deceased, permission to carry on with life for the bereaved or setting in motion the transition of the dead to another level of life or existence. Funeral rituals tend to form part of people's solidarity within a family, community or even society. When viewed from this perspective, it is logical to conclude that funerals are a powerful means of bringing people closer to each other and allowing life to go on after death. This kind of ritual or ceremony is perceived as forming the functional part of funerals. Obviously, there is another side to this argument: if the funeral ritual should fail to serve its intended purpose, the outcome may be seen as dysfunctional and expensive, with long-lasting negative impact on the bereaved.

Funerals and their rituals are seen as the last act of showing respect for the dead and internalising him or her into the memory of the living. Internalisation allows for synergy of emotional activity to occur (which is contrary to the teachings of Freud); that is, the bereaved carries on with his or her life and can invest in others, while simultaneously investing his or her energy in the deceased person. Internalisation allows the bereaved to choose when to remember their dead and when to get on with their lives. These are real choices at difficult times, and the bereaved would be left guilt-free because they have the opportunity to attend to both the deceased and their own life. This would also ensure a healthier state of mind for the bereaved and a return to some kind of social normality for them. Death should not result in emotional imprisonment for the bereaved. It is important for theorist and now practitioners to be more sensitive to human feelings and allow the uniqueness of that individual (particularly when bereaved) to flourish. The bereaved would benefit more from less theoretical entrapments and be helped according to their identified needs. This point, and similar others, will be developed in the next chapter, where arguments are made to move away from staged theories and 'tick box approaches' to bereavement care. There is obviously a great need now for us all to *listen* to what the patient or bereaved really want. As professionals we can play our part in making dying, death and bereavement more personal and less difficult an experience to negotiate.

References

Appleyard B. (1999) Death of a dream. *Sunday Times*, Books, p. 4, 7 March.

Bayliss, J. (1996) *Understanding Loss and Grief*. National Extension College Trust, Cambridge.

Bee, H. (1994) *Lifespan Development*. HarperCollins, New York.

Bertman, S. L. (1979) *Facing Death. Images, Insights and Interventions*. Hampshere Publishing Corporation, New York.

Black, D. (1978) The bereaved child. *Journal of Child Psychology and Psychiatry*, **19**, 278–92.

Clark, D. (ed.) (1996) *The Sociology of Death*. Blackwell, Oxford.

Denison, K. (1999) The theology and liturgy of funerals: a view from the church of Wales. *Mortality*, **4**(1), 63–74.

Durkheim, E. (1954) *The Elementary Forms of Religious Life*. Allen and Unwin, London.

Frazer, J. G. (1968) *In Man, God, and Immortality: Thoughts on Human Progress*. Trinity College Press, Cambridge.

Fulton, R. (1995) Contemporary funeral practices. In: *Successful Funeral Service Practice* (ed. H. C. Raether). Prentice Hall, Englewood Cliffs, NJ.

Jackson, E. (1978) *The Many Faces of Grief*. SCM.

Kolakowski, L. (1983) The mummy's tomb. *New Republic*, 4 July.

Leming, M. R. and Dickinson, G. E. (1998) *Understanding Death, Dying and Bereavement*, 4th edn. Harcourt Brace, Philadelphia.

Littlewood, J. (1993) The denial of death and rites of passage in contemporary societies. In: *The Sociology of Death* (ed. D. Clark). Blackwell Science, Oxford.

Long, G. (1987) Organisations and identity: obituaries 1856–1972. *Social Forces*, **65**(4), 964–1001.

Mandelbaum, D. (1959) Social uses of funeral rites. In: *The Meaning of Death* (ed. H. Feifel). McGraw-Hill, New York.

Malinowski, B. (1984) Death and the reintegration of a group. In: *Magic, Science and Religion and Other Essays* (ed. B. Malinowski). Doubleday, New York.

Prior, L. (1989) *The Social Organisation of Death. Medical Discourse and Social Practices in Belfast*. Macmillan, London.

Rees, D. (1997) *Death and Bereavement. The Psychological, Religious and Cultural Interfaces*, Chapter 5. Whurr, London.

Seale, C. (1998) *Constructing Death. The Sociology of Dying and Bereavement*. Cambridge University Press, Cambridge.

Sheatsley, P. B. and Feldman, J. J. (1964) The assassination of President Kennedy: a preliminary report on public relations and behavior. *Public Opinion Quarterly*. **28**, 189–215.

Sudnow, D. (1967) *Passing On: The Social Organisation of Dying*. Prentice Hall, Englewood Cliffs, NJ.

Van Gennep, A. (1961) *The Rites of Passage*. University of Chicago, Chicago.

Walter, T. (1997) *The Revival of Death*. Routledge, London.

CHAPTER 11

Rethinking loss and grief

Jean Bayliss

This book has presented a range of perspectives on death and dying. The unique experiencing of dying and bereavement has been viewed through a prism, reflecting and refracting the light of insight from a variety of angles. Throughout the book there is an awareness that however many facets of the prism are explored and however many general principles can be shared and agreed, the experiencing of dying and death is uniquely individual. As a patient once said to me after having been told by a variety of people (some of them professionals) that he was 'going through the grieving process':

> Why don't they forget their theories – I am the one who's dying, and it's happening here, not in a book

This chapter, then, is written from a personal perspective and aims to sum up the views expressed in the book by focusing on the need to value the theory, but keep the individual in mind. This approach may be a step toward making dying less difficult for the individual. The personal perspectives have arisen from several sources: counselling practice, clinical supervision, training others in understanding and working with loss and grief, personal experience and a growing concern that the received wisdom about the so-called 'grieving process' did not seem to accurately describe what many grieving people were experiencing. Indeed, it was an angry outburst by a young bereaved father of three which first prompted me to look again at what actually seems to be real for grieving people. He declared:

> I am *not* in a process – this isn't like a can of beans on a conveyor belt!

and

> I don't think I'm *going* anywhere, unless it's round in circles.

The work of Julie Ann Wambach (1985) has confirmed that there seems to be a fixed belief in *a* 'grieving process' and my own research suggests that many helpers and counsellors also think that *a* process exists and that it is, for the most part, linear. Grieving people, it is suggested, go through stages or phases or work at tasks. Whilst these formulations may well be true and helpful for some people to be aware of, my concern is that they may be used prescriptively, rather than descriptively.

The valuable pioneering work of Elizabeth Kübler-Ross (1970) gave us a model of what may happen in grief. Her model of Denial, Anger, Bargaining, Depression and Acceptance has been consistently used in terminal care training and is sometimes used to describe bereavement grief (George, 1992).

It seems unlikely that someone with the vision and humanity of Kübler-Ross would have expected dying (or bereaved) people to march obligingly through these five stages in order; yet the model is frequently used very rigidly. Occasionally, too, an aura of disapproval seems to exist around those who 'get stuck' in one or other of the stages, or who (tiresomely?) stay 'in denial'. I have myself supported an oncology nurse who was under considerable pressure because 'You're not getting them through to acceptance quickly enough'. The concept of 'Acceptance' seems itself to have gained mythic proportions as of an almost beatific state – which is not how Kübler-Ross herself defined the final stage anyway. The more recent adaptation of the Kübler-Ross model also has a linear feel to it:

- Shock
- Denial (not disbelief)
- Anger
- Guilt
- Fear
- Anxiety
- Despair/depression
- Acceptance/resignation

Indeed, while I have seen in dying persons isolation, envy, bargaining, depression, and acceptance, I do not believe that these are necessarily 'stages' of the dying process, and I am not all convinced that they are lived through in that order, or, for that matter, in any universal order.

What I do see is complicated clustering of intellectual and affective states, some fleeting, lasting for a moment or a day or a week, set not unexpectedly against the backdrop of that person's total personality, his 'philosophy of life' (Schneidman, 1977)

In similar fashion, thanatologist Mansell Pattison states:

I find *no* evidence... to support specific stages of dying. Rather, dying patients demonstrate a wide variety of emotions that ebb and flow throughout our entire life as we face conflicts and crises. It does seem misleading, then, to search for and determine stages of dying.

Rather, I suggest that our task is to determine the stresses and crises at a specific time, to respond to the emotions generated by that issue, and, in essence, to *respond to where the patient is at* in his or her living-dying.

We do not make the patient conform to our idealised concept of dying but respond to the patient's actual dying experience (Wass, 1988)

Why is it, I wondered, that helpers adopt these models (sometimes, perhaps, without reference to their original formulations)? Why do we prefer a model, rather than accepting that grieving people are living people who 'do their own thing'? My thoughts were summed up by Dee Cooper (1991), a research assistant writing 17 years after the death of her son:

I suspect that stage models and frameworks of grief and words like resolution have more to do with professionals containing their anxieties than reality

It may also be that when confronted with the chaos of experiencing emotional, cognitive, behavioural and physical dimensions that we call 'grief' we distance ourselves by applying a model, because the *model* feels safer than the chaos.

Although his model is not especially new, it is interesting that Weisman's model of an *appropriate death* has not gained the status of the linear models of dying (Weisman, 1984). The model offers carers, whether professionals or not, a challenge to achieve with and for a dying person a death that is appropriate to his or her unique experience. It may be significant that Weisman avoids the term 'good' death, with all the controversy which that arouses. He suggests that we aim to help a dying person in four areas:

- Reducing conflict
- Enabling a death which is compatible with their views of themselves and their achievements
- Preserving or restoring relationships
- Fulfilling some of the dying person's expressed aims

In some senses these may seem like modest aims, but they are active and require a strong commitment to communication. Most of all they require *us* to *engage actively* with the dying person, rather than approaching them with

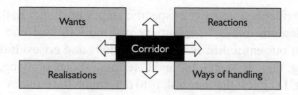

Figure 11.1 The four-room model (Prunkl and Berry, 1989).

a predetermined set of stages that they may be 'in' and feeling helpless when they are not.

In an attempt to develop a non-linear model, Prunkl and Berry (1989) considered how the dying (or grieving) person may – like the rest of us – change almost from minute to minute, and handle a variety of stimuli both external and internal in a variety of ways. They offer us their four-room model (Figure 11.1).

They asked helpers to reflect that, if the 'house' is seen three-dimensionally, a person may move between each of the 'rooms' almost continually – or rest in one for a while. They found no evidence that stages occurred. The different rooms represented changing emotions and situations (for example 'realisations, wants, reactions and ways of handling') as the person moved and crossed the corridors.

A circular model was suggested to me by a patient of my own who saw his grief much more as 'swinging about' (Figure 11.2).

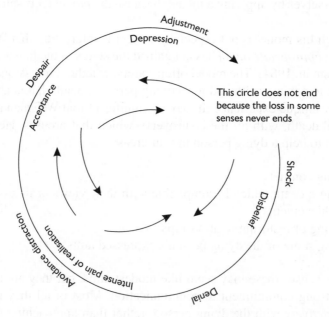

Figure 11.2 A circular model of grief.

If we are to help people facing the imminent loss of all that is dear to them and the loss of life itself, perhaps we need to examine more closely why we cling to formulations which may well distance us from people and equally may well not reflect or resonate with what is actually happening for the person. Perhaps we should 'forget order and work with chaos'.

Terms like 'grief work', and 'working through' have almost become the *lingua franca* of bereavement and seem to have become separated from their original psychodynamic and psychoanalytical contexts, rather as 'the grieving process' seems to be regarded as fact. The questions I found myself asking about the bereaved clients/patients I try to help was what exactly *is* 'grief work' (now that it no longer has Freud's theory attached to it)? Is my client really 'working *through*'? It often seems more as if she or he is working *at*. And 'which process?' – is it tasks, stages, phases (how many?).

There has recently been a significant groundswell of thinking which challenges linear or sequential models of grief, whilst acknowledging that their framework can be helpful to some people sometimes. The concern is more that a too rigid adherence to any model can mean that a grieving person who does not, obligingly, go through 'the process' may be seen as 'abnormal'. There is anxiety that grief, the natural reaction to loss, can in this way be pathologised. The sequential models which have, perhaps, had most influence on bereavement counselling/therapy are those of Worden (1991) and Parkes (1986), both of which come from a psychodynamic root. Worden's Tasks of Grief model suggests that the bereaved 'work through' a series of tasks to resolve their grief. The tasks were, originally:

- To accept the reality of the loss
- To experience the pain of grief
- To adjust to an environment no longer containing the loved one
- To reinvest emotion

The final task has been adjusted to 'to relocate the lost one' in order to move on with life, Worden's revision seeming to mean that rather than reinvesting the emotions and hopes originally invested in the deceased (a Freudian concept), the bereaved work to find a new place in their emotional lives for the deceased. This model had been offered to the young father I quoted at the start of this chapter, who said, of the first three 'tasks' that 'to have done any of that *in order* would have been a luxury' and five years after his wife's death he often found himself disbelieving the reality that she was no longer with him, yet he was functioning well and in no sense could be seen as grieving abnormally.

Parkes' model of:

- Numbness
- Searching and yearning

- Disorganisation
- Reorganisation

described by Rubin (1996) as a 'pathway' along which the bereaved 'progress', is also widely used and was the initial training model for CRUSE, the national Bereavement Care Charity. It may be that the notion of 'progress' is one of the reasons why there are increasing challenges to a sequential view of grief. 'Progress' implies that those who move along the pathway are somehow 'doing well' and, more worryingly, that those who do not grieve in any ordered way are somehow, as one respondent in my own research put it, 'not trying to work through the stages of grief'. There has for some time been a movement away from setting time boundaries for the stages (amazingly, in the 1940s – perhaps because of the war – Lindemann (1944) proposed 'recovery' over four to six weeks!), but there is still some sense that grief should in some way be time limited if it is 'normal'. This seems to be linked to the *necessity* of experiencing (or working through) painful feelings in order to 'let go' – another common term in the language of bereavement. If the bereaved either do not experience those feelings intensely or if the feelings persist, grief is often labelled as 'abnormal' and may be pathologised (see Raphael, 1983, pp. 59–60). The work of Wortmann and Silver (1989) is especially challenging to these formulations of bereavement grief. They suggest that there is a contradiction somewhere at the heart of the theory. Their research did not find universal evidence of the extreme distress or depression which Bowlby (1981) and others have seen as virtually essential for 'healthy' grieving; nor did they find that those who did not exhibit intense grief reactions could be said to be denying it, or 'in denial' – rather the reverse. The contradiction they cite is the popular belief that those who do not experience the pain intensely will, at some later point, suffer problematic reactions. If this were so, those who *do* experience intense pain should – logically – adapt better to their bereavement. Yet the opposite seems to be true – those most distressed early on (i.e. who have experienced the pain of grief, Worden's Task Two) are *more*, not less, likely to be depressed later on. They say:

> The data clearly suggests that 'absent grief' is not necessarily problematic, ... delayed grief is far less common than clinical lore would suggest.

They suggest that there is little empirical evidence that not 'working through' tasks or stages will lead to what one worried client once described to me as, 'a fear that it will sneak up on me and get me when I don't expect it' because her grief was not going along the recommended route! Wortmann and Silver (1989) also challenge any notion of time-limited grief. Parkes and Weiss (1983) themselves were surprised at the ongoing grief of widows, but

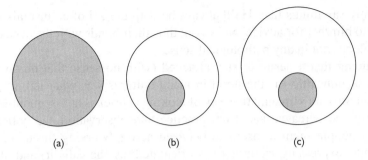

(a)   (b)   (c)

Figure 11.3 Growing around grief model (Tonkin, 1996).

Wortmann and Silver see it as normal and concur with the experience of Dee Cooper, quoted earlier, that grief does not follow a fixed pattern in time or in intensity.

Some interesting work in this respect has come from a study of bereaved people in New Zealand. The findings of this study by Tonkin (1996) can be represented graphically as shown in Figure 11.3. Soon after the bereavement the grieving person felt 'all loss' (Figure 11.3(a)), and it was predicted that over time the grief would diminish, whilst the person would remain, as it were, the 'same size' (Figure 11.3(b)). Yet what happened over time was that the grief stayed the same size, but the person grew round it (Figure 11.3(c)).

This confirms the experience of many I have counselled who report a strengthening of themselves, and an enlargement of their understanding of themselves and of their compassion for others. This is not to say that some grief is not exceptionally complex and complicated, but that to label grief as 'pathological' because it does not conform to models may well be to deny the positive effects it can have.

The strong influence of Bowlby's attachment theory has also led to some rethinking of bereavement grief. The view that for a healthy adjustment to a bereavement to take place the bonds of attachment need to be broken, in particular, has been contested. Tony Walter (1996) concurs with the research carried out by Silverman and Nickman (1996) that, far from detaching from the deceased, the bereaved retain very strong attachments, although the relationship and dynamics of the attachment change over time. In *Bereavement and Biography* Walter points out how an event like the funeral can enlarge and extend our understanding of the deceased, thus changing the nature of the relationship. He also points to the need that the bereaved feel to talk about the deceased – in the linear formulations this might be seen as coping with denial or checking the reality of the loss, but Walter sees it more as building the new relationship with the dead. We can, in a sense, all be our own researchers here in thinking about how we still relate to those who have had a significant role in our lives. I am well aware of my tendency to 'check out' how my parents might react to or value events in my own life, for instance. Bereaved people frequently say things like 'He'll always be with me', 'I often just talk to her', 'I look to him/her for advice' and so on; thus their bonds with the deceased are renewed, but not in any pathological sense.

Noticing that a desire to stay attached (with no sense that this might be morbid or unhealthy) is the norm in many cultures was what led, in part, to Margaret Stroebe's imaginative way of looking at grief as non-sequential. From diaries of the bereaved and from practice and observation she noticed that grieving people seem to oscillate between active 'working through', breaking bonds, expressing feelings (loss orientated, as she calls it) and allowing themselves, on the other hand, to be distracted, to take on new roles and take up new activities (restorative). (See also Figure 11.4, showing the dual process model of coping with grief.) Stroebe does not dispute that some aspects of the sequential models may well be real, but that they are not experienced in any kind of order, but more in the way that we deal with any of life's stresses, by sometimes confronting them and sometimes 'putting them on the back burner', as one teenager described his grief to me after the death of his sister.

Western theories of grief and models of bereavement

Western theories and models of bereavement, grief and mourning have, to a great extent, been based on Freud's *Mourning and Melancholia*, in which he asks the question, 'Why should this [the process he saw as mourning] be so painful?'. His colleague Melanie Klein attempted to answer the question and it is her theories which are influencing the groundswell of opinion that a linear process of grieving may not be real for some people. Klein is best known for her work with children, from which she drew her theory of 'internalising' – that is, that from infancy humans develop an ability to internalise the person they love by keeping an inner sense of the presence of those close to them. For Klein this person was almost always likely to be the mother, who the baby was in time able to realise went away and returned by keeping an image of her, so much so that that it becomes part of the baby's 'self', and the infant is able to hold the image as comfort and not be distressed by the mother's absence, as long is it is not too prolonged. Klein's theory thus explains how grief involves rebuilding an inner self when the loved person has died. The feeling of 'internalising' is well expressed by the famous author Daphne du Maurier:

> ... if you go away, if you travel, even if you decide to make your home elsewhere, the spirit of tenderness, of love, will not desert you. You will find that it has become part of you, rising from within yourself... death the last enemy has been overcome.

This experience of 'internalising' the deceased is frequently expressed by the bereaved in terms such as, 'I know s/he will always be with me', which are the very opposite of 'letting go' or of 'moving on'.

Klein's theory was developed to include what are called 'transitional objects'. Young children frequently keep with them a piece of cloth or a soft toy which causes great distress if it is lost (or perhaps removed for hygiene reasons!). The theory suggests that these objects are associated by the child with the security of the mother-figure (hence the term comfort blanket) and form a transition between her and independence. In the same way, in adult grief, an object is treasured because it is a comforting link with the deceased. Many bereaved partners disclose how they sleep with the dead person's dressing gown, and – sadly – often think that they will be criticised for this, but Klein's theory reassures us that it is a normal human reaction to loss and can be a healthy part of rebuilding the inner self, as she said:

> The pain felt in the slow process... in the work of mourning thus seems to be partly due to the necessity not only to renew the links to the external world and thus continuously to re-experience the loss, but at the same time... to rebuild with anguish the inner world which is felt to be in danger of deteriorating and collapsing.

Learning difficulties

The pain of loss for people with learning difficulties is an under researched – indeed until relatively recently an unacknowledged – area. Thankfully, it is increasingly recognised that people with learning difficulties experience grief and that not being able, or in some cases not being 'allowed' to express it can lead to problems with behaviour and other unhappy outcomes. The (true) narrative of 'John' will serve as an example of how imperative it is to recognise and respect grief in those with a learning difficulty.

> John was in his late thirties when his father died. He was an only child, lovingly cared for by elderly parents and very affectionate. He attended a day centre/workshop where he took great pride in the tasks he had learned to perform. His mother told the day centre staff about the bereavement and that John had attended the funeral, but that she was unsure how fully he understood the significance of the death or whether he fully grasped that it was permanent. The staff devised a very sensitive programme, based on missing, loss, funerals, remembering and included the whole group. John was given lots of attention and many

of his fellow students gave hugs or presents as signs of sympathy and affection.

Very unexpectedly, John's mother also died within a short space of time. As there was no one to care for him at home he was found a place in a residential setting, where his background was not known and which was not close to the day centre, which he was no longer able to attend.

His mother's death was not explained to him and no rituals of mourning were observed. John's behaviour deteriorated: he became very introverted, his language skills regressed and his general responsiveness declined.

Maureen Oswin, who cared for her sister who had a learning disability until her sister died has written movingly about the difficulties both she, as carer, and her sister experienced. Some of these were to do with benefits and other practical help during the terminal phase of her sister's illness and some to do with the insurmountable problem of accessing palliative care.

Her writing and subsequent research are a reminder that our theories of death and dying need to be inclusive. We often use the term 'inclusive' or 'inclusion' to mean culturally or even racially inclusive and certainly theory should show awareness in these areas, but we need too to reflect on how excluded those with learning difficulties are from the growth in interest in palliative care and in bereavement.

Materialism and the experience of grief

We have noted that many of the theories and models of bereavement are Eurocentric. The West has grown steadily wealthier in the 20th and 21st centuries. At the same time poverty in other parts of the world appears to have remained static or to have worsened. The HIV/AIDS pandemic, the terrible effects of the Asian tsunami, and the continuing starvation of whole populations all highlight the need for some understanding of the loss and grief experienced by those in abject poverty. There is currently much research into 'happiness' – what makes us happy? One conclusion seems to be that the increased wealth in the West has coincided with a *de*crease in happiness. This perhaps begins to explain the growing interest in dying, death and bereavement.

It as if we in the West are unable to accept that death is as much a part of our lives as it is of the poorest, and that whatever we do, we are mortal. This may be a very inspiring area for study if it helps us to be more aware of our universal common humanity.

Loss-oriented   **Restoration-oriented**

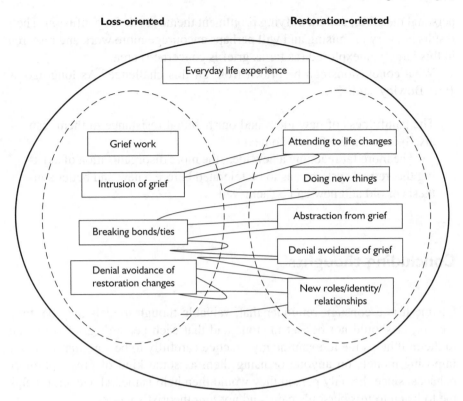

Figure 11.4 A dual process model of coping with grief (Stroebe and Schutt, 1995).

Finally, it is evident that many of the symptoms of depression are very similar to some of the manifestations of grief. Cognitive behavioural therapy is one of the few counselling/psychotherapy interventions which offers itself for rigorous evaluation and which seems to be particularly successful with clinical and reactive depression. It would then seem sensible to use cognitive behavioural techniques to help grieving people, yet most counselling seems to focus on the affective aspects of grief, urging the grieving person to express or 'work through' a range of powerful feelings. Grief is, of course, very powerful in the feelings it evokes, but it is also experienced cognitively, physically and behaviourally. Perhaps as helpers we need to focus on these areas too? To date there is little work in this field, but one interesting piece of research (Powers and Wampold, 1994) suggests that focus on cognitive behavioural factors could be of great help to grieving people. Grief is, in a sense, the greatest stressor most of us will experience and perhaps we can learn from techniques of stress management, which are, mainly, cognitive behavioural. Powers and Wampold attempted the techniques, for example, differentiating devaluing the deceased and attending to life tasks; engaging in health promotion; attributing personal meaning; and identifying prominent themes to assist confusion. Their results are very promising and will perhaps encourage more work and research in this largely unexplored (as far as grief is concerned) area.

What conclusions can be drawn from all this challenge? As long ago as 1961 Bowlby said:

> The painfulness of new ideas and our habitual resistance to them, can also be seen in the (grief) context.
>
> The more far reaching a new idea, the more disorganisation of existing theoretical systems has to be tolerated before a new and better synthesis of old and new can be achieved

Concluding thoughts

For me it is a constant reminder that, valuable though models may be, they are not, or should not be, set in stone and that each person's grief is unique to them. It helps me to examine my practice carefully to be sure that I am not imposing models on anyone or using them as some kind of prescription or panacea, since the only person they would then help is me. Above all, it helps me to listen to *this* person's pain, and not *that* theorist's model.

Dying and death bring very sharply into focus the profound questions, 'Who am I?' and 'What makes me, me?'. The imminent loss of self, and for the bereaved, the loss of who the deceased was, can be the most disturbing aspects of loss and their very nature means that they are rarely addressed by carers either professionally or informally. The sense that we cannot answer these questions for ourselves may make us wary of exploring existential or spiritual issues with the dying or bereaved. This apparent deficit is perhaps why we need models as a defence. Maybe we should follow Jung's advice:

> Learn your theories as well as you can, but put them aside when you touch the Miracle of the living Soul. Not theories, but your own creative individuality must decide.

References

Bowlby, J. (1961) Processes of mourning. *International Journal of Psychoanalysis,* **42**, 317–40.

Bowlby, J. (1981) Psychoanalysis as natural science. *International Review of Psychoanalysis*, **82**, 243–55.

Cooper, D. (1991) Long-term grief. *British Medical Journal*, **303**.

George, H. (1992) *Psychological Support In Death and Dying*. Resurgam, Reading.

Jackson, E. N. (1957) *Understanding Grief*. Abingdon Press, Nashville, TN.

Kübler-Ross, E. (1970) *On Death and Dying*. Tavistock, New York.

Lindemann, E. (1944) The symptomatology and management of acute grief. *American Journal of Psychiatry*, **101**.

Parkes, C. M. (1986) *Bereavement: Studies of Grief in Adult Life*. Penguin, London.

Parkes, C. M. and Weiss, R. (1983) *Recovery From Bereavement*. Basic Books, New York.

Pincus, L. (1974) *Death and the Family. Management Of Acute Grief*. Pantheon Books, New York.

Powers, L. E. and Wampold, B. E. (1994) Cognitive behavioural factors in adjustment to adult bereavement. *Death Studies*, **181**.

Prunkl, P. R. and Berry, R. L. (1989) *Death Week*. Hemisphere Publishing, New York.

Raphael, B. (1983) *An Anatomy of Bereavement*. Hutchinson, London.

Rubin, S. (1996) *Continuing Bonds*. Taylor & Francis, London.

Shneidman, E. S. (1977) Aspects of the dying process. *Psychiatric Annals*, **8**, 25–40.

Silverman, P. R. and Nickman, S. L. (1996) *Continuing Bonds*. Taylor & Francis, Philadelphia.

Stroebe, M. (1992) Coping with bereavement. *Omega*, **261**.

Stroebe, M. S. and Schutt, H. (1995) Helping the bereaved come to terms with loss. In: *Bereavement and Counselling*. St George's Mental Health Sciences, London.

Tonkin, L. (1996) *Bereavement Care*, **15**(1), 10.

Walter, T. (1996) A new model for grief, bereavement and biography. *Mortality*, **1**, 7–25.

Wambuch, J. A. (1985) The grief process as a social construct. *Omega*, **163**.

Wass, H. (ed.) (1988) *Dying: Facing the Facts*. Taylor & Francis, Washington.

Weisman, A. (1984) *The Coping Capacity*. Human Sciences, New York.

Worden, J. W. (1991) *Grief Counselling and Grief Therapy*. Springer, New York.

Wortmann, C. and Silver, R. (1989) The myths of coping with loss. *Journal of Counselling and Clinical Psychology*, **57**(3), 349–57.

CHAPTER 12

The last word

Brian Nyatanga

This second edition, like the first, has continued to explore the challenging question, 'Why is it so difficult to die?'. This has proved a difficult question to answer, but also not one that many people take time to ponder about openly. Even in today's societies, with increased terrorist attacks and murders, most people choose to focus on other aspects of life, at a conscious level anyway, but not always on death and dying. We all know and accept that death will happen to us at some point, but somehow we find it the most difficult topic to engage in. In a way, perhaps we think that by not talking about death, we may somehow magically avert it. However, there seems to be some interesting ironies when you consider how people behave towards their own death. One is found in those who choose to plan and prepare for their own death privately by purchasing insurance and funeral packages, and yet feel unable to discuss their death openly. We also know that there is now a plethora of literature and information on death and dying, but that too does not seem to overtly change our attitude to and perceptions of death.

Many readers, friends and colleagues have asked me why I chose the title *Why is it So Difficult to Die?* for this book. The simple answer is that there is no evidence, for me, to suggest the contrary. Up to now there is no overwhelming evidence to persuade me to believe that dying (particularly in Western societies) is an easy thing to do. Despite the advances in medical technology and the availability of euthanasia (see Chapter 7), dying remains a difficult 'thing' to do. Even with regard to the anticipated and 'accepted' death, the actual point of death itself seems to provoke different emotions and reactions, including anger and sadness. Throughout this book, all contributors have tried to shed some light on how to explain this phenomenon and why it is difficult to negotiate. The focus on the concepts of death, euthanasia, and ethical and medical perspectives was aimed at offering possible explanations of dying from different perspectives.

I truly believe that the additional information in this second edition has helped in some way towards our understanding of this difficult concept. I also hope that all the chapters have raised our thinking to another level, which should help in our teaching, researching and philosophising about death. The medicalisation of death and its drawbacks will have made you think about how medical intervention eases the difficulty of dying. The discussion around medicalisation of death has been frank and has highlighted some of the problems that medicine faces in palliative care provision. It may seem strange to have medical intervention in palliative care settings, bearing in mind that historically it was poor-quality medical care of the dying patients that prompted the creation of palliative care. I must stress here, as a way of reassuring the few heretics out there, that the type of medical input we see in palliative care is very different from that which most people criticise in hospitals. We have palliative medicine which in my opinion offers a different type of care that views the patient as a person with cancer, and not just organs with a disease. The arguments on medicalisation of dying have been well articulated by Gannon in Chapters 4 and 5. We need medicine, nursing and the therapies to work together towards the benefit and comfort of the patient. In working together it is important that we acknowledge the different professional memories we each hold about the patients we look after. It is quite possible for professionals to end up with different professional memories about the same patient. This only helps to emphasise the individual differences in how each professional approaches, negotiates and deals with a patient's experiences. What is important in acknowledging these different professional memories is that we can all try to reconcile these memories to achieve a much better quality of life for the dying patient.

Equally, the ethical considerations needed to arrive at 'the right decision' are important and in most cases always challenging. There is no one ethical paradigm to follow and that in itself poses dilemmas when making decisions at the end of life. However, decisions still have to be made whilst dealing with the patient's constantly changing condition and needs. For professionals faced with making decisions every day, there is a propensity to feel guilty if a decision results in a negative outcome. It would therefore be unfortunate if professionals ended up feeling this way, because most professionals are genuine and honest when making such difficult and complex decisions. I therefore still believe in the philosophy I was taught on entering palliative care all those years ago: the decision you make is *right* at the time of making it. The importance of holding on to such a view is that, in making any decision, we tend to use all our senses. What we see, feel, hear and many more things about the patient are crucial guides to what decisions we make, in addition to the clinical picture. If someone else were to talk to (assess) the same patient 10 or so minutes later they might make a different decision from yours, but this might be because the situation before them is different from that which you experienced. Using a philosophy like mine may mean that we do not feel so guilty after each decision we make, because all decisions in palliative care tend to be difficult, but they must be right at the time we make them.

If we consider death for a citizen of the Netherlands, where euthanasia is legalised, the actual process of dying is not necessarily easy for that dying patient, his family or the attending physician. Chapter 7 discussed the process of euthanasia, and at the end de Vocht concluded that even with the knowledge that euthanasia is possible and freely available, dying itself does not suddenly become an easy thing to do. What then would make dying easy, particularly when we all know it will happen to each one of us at some point? Maybe I am being optimistic in thinking that dying should be easy.

Would the knowledge that one has a choice of ending one's life itself help ease the anxieties and fears of dying? Maybe if we had not known what it is to be alive, it would be easy to face our own death. In this case being alive assumes having a life that is enjoyable and that one is satisfied and happy to want to hold on to 'dear life'. If life were not all these positive things, one would find it hard to see the need to hold on to it. It is also true that even those who may not see any positive aspects in their own life would not necessarily choose to end it. They might wish to be alive for their family and probably children and grandchildren. In other words, the focus changes from themselves to others.

One would have thought that those with a belief in life after death would find dying easy, but that again is not always the case. One wonders therefore whether viewing death as a transition to another life is somehow a psychological buffer to our own fear of death. It appears the more death remains unpredictable and indiscriminate, the less people understand it and therefore it will continue to be difficult to accommodate it. In that case dying will also remain a difficult thing to do. It is probably the basis of what some commentators now consider to be the core of existential death anxiety (Greenberg *et al.*, 2004). The knowledge of our being non-existent is itself powerful trigger of death anxiety. If this assertion is acceptable, it would suggest that being alive is synonymous with death anxiety (Heidegger, 1962). The first assertion about the nature of anxiety is that, anxiety is the state in which a person is aware of his or her possible non-being or non-existence. In other words, our mere existence is in itself sufficient to create existential anxiety in most people with an awareness of death. According to Tillich (1952), 'existential' in this context means that it is not the abstract knowledge of non-being which produces anxiety but the awareness that non-being is a part of one's own being. It is not the realisation of universal transitions, nor even the experience of the death of others, but the impression of these events on the always latent awareness of our own having to die that produces anxiety.

In summary, the advances in symptom control (both physical and psycho-emotional) go a long way in easing the pain and suffering of those who are dying. I believe that health care professionals working with dying patients perceive themselves as privileged to be in such a special role supporting and helping the patient achieve his or her own unique death. They are also privileged to share special social intercourse with the dying on both the physical and psychological levels. However, there is a potential 'price to pay' for such intimacy. We have to recognise that doing this type of work day in, day out, has its own emotional toll on the professionals; and that is why it is important for employing organisations to ensure that social support like clinical supervision is readily available to all professionals. It is important in caring and palliative care in particular to provide such support before a crisis happens, as this affords professionals the time and space needed to be prepared for difficult situations. Support should therefore be seen as a preventive measure from possible burnout. Support for health care professionals also means minimising cost by reducing burnout-related absenteeism.

Finally, it is my hope that this book has provided you with something new to think about with reference to the ever-present but complex notion of death and dying. It is important that we continue to understand patients' needs, whilst caring for them and their families and helping them to achieve a unique death that reflects their own individuality and priorities. I believe that would be a worthwhile legacy to leave behind in palliative care.

References

Greenberg, J., Koole, S. L. and Pyszczynski, T. (eds.) (2004) *Handbook of Experimental Existential Pyschology*. The Guildford Press, New York.

Heidegger, M. (1962) *Being and Time*. Blackwell, Oxford

Tillich, P. (1952) *The Courage to Be*. Yale University Press, New Haven.

Twycross, R. (1994) *Introducing Palliative Care*. Radcliffe Medical Press, Oxford.

Vachon, M. (2000) Burnout and symptoms of stress in staff working in palliative care. In: *Handbook of Psychiatry in Palliative Medicine* (eds. H. Chochinov and W. Breitbart). Oxford University Press, Oxford.

Index